Ties of Distinc[tion]

Introduction by Christopher Sells

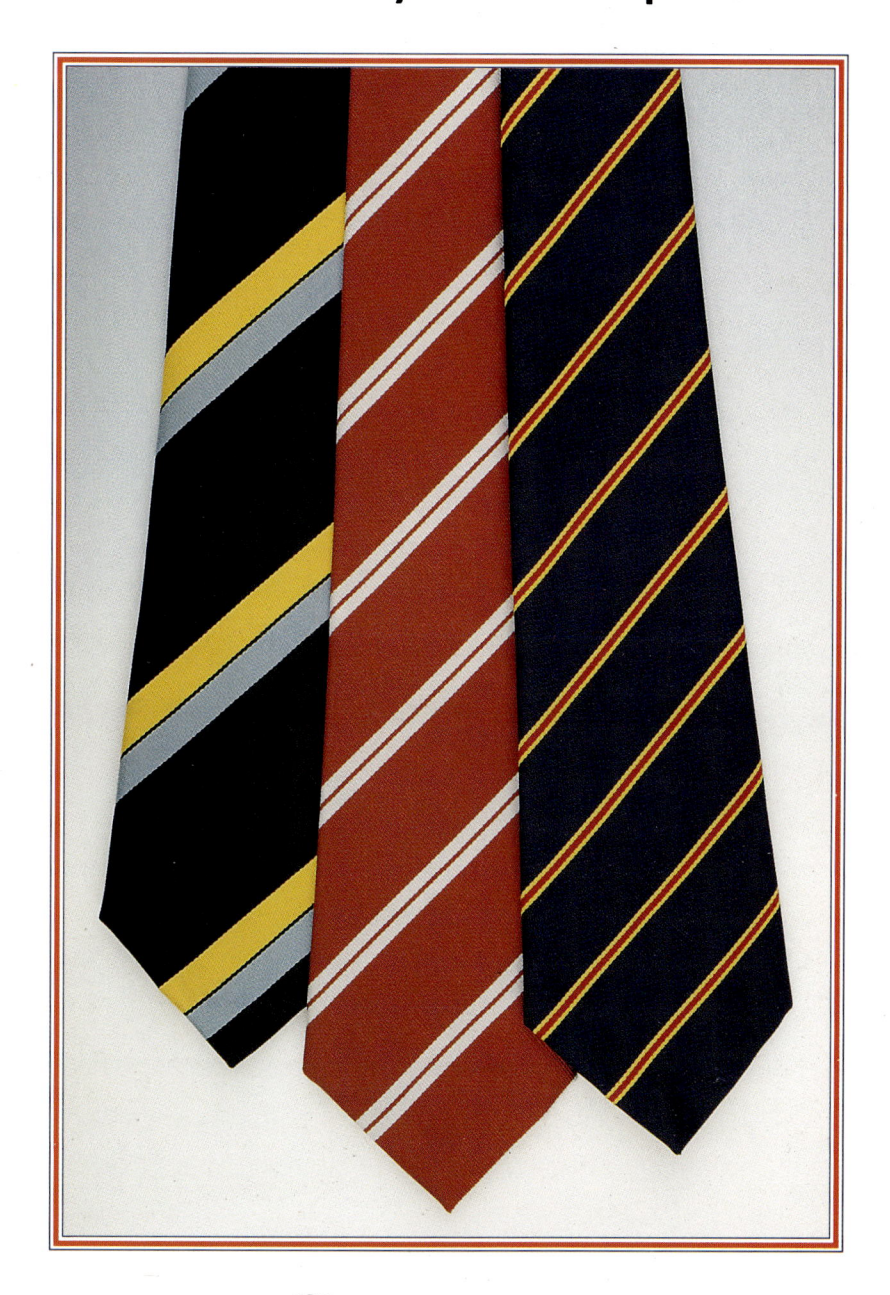

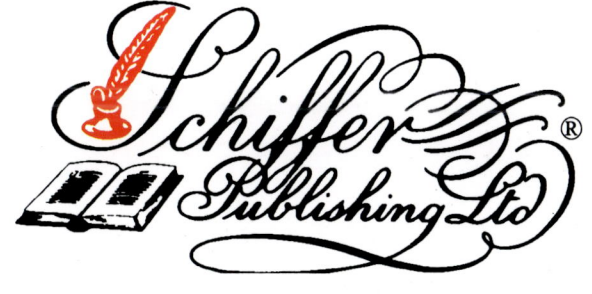

Schiffer Publishing Ltd

4880 Lower Valley Road, Atglen, PA 19310 USA

Copyright © 1998 by Schiffer Publishing Ltd.
Library of Congress Catalog Card Number: 98-85949

All rights reserved. No part of this work may be reproduced or used in any form or by any means—graphic, electronic, or mechanical, including photocopying or information storage and retrieval systems—without written permission from the copyright holder.
"Schiffer," "Schiffer Publishing Ltd. & Design," and the "Design of pen and ink well" are registered trademarks of Schiffer Publishing, Ltd.

Designed By Bonnie M. Hensley
Typeset in Zurich Blk BT/Zurich BT

ISBN: 0-7643-0633-2
Printed in China

Published by Schiffer Publishing Ltd.
4880 Lower Valley Road
Atglen, PA 19310
Phone: (610) 593-1777; Fax: (610) 593-2002
E-mail: Schifferbk@aol.com
Please write for a free catalog.
This book may be purchased from the publisher.
Please include $3.95 for shipping.

In Europe Schiffer books are distributed by
Bushwood Books
6 Marksbury Avenue Kew Gardens
Surrey TW9 4JF England
Phone: 44 (0) 181 392-8585; Fax: 44 (0) 181 392-9876
E-mail: Bushwd@aol.com

Please try your bookstore first.

We are interested in hearing from authors
with book ideas on related subjects.

Contents

Introduction 4
Royal Armoured Corps—Cavalry 5
Regiments and Yeomanry 15
Gurkha, Indian, and Colonial 45
Naval 61
Royal Marines 66
Air Force 68
Universities 73
London Colleges, Medical Schools 78
Oxford Colleges 83
Old Boys 89
Clubs, etc. 99
National and County Ties 103

Introduction

I like regimental ties. They are bold, sober, gay, forthright, vigorous designs, evocative things full of resonance for those who recognize them and, for those who don't, nonetheless recognizably serious items of clothing. These ties do not imply a moment of vanity in front of the bathroom mirror after the morning shave. In Britain, a striped tie which is not a regimental tie is an old school tie, a club tie, or a college tie. If none of these, it is a solecism: no manufacturer in Britain would find it worthwhile to promote a striped tie as a nice thing to wear for its own sake.

We have all of us known, since our first day at school, that this thing around our necks is not for decoration, but to define us, to others and to ourselves. It makes us one of a group, for better or worse. We will wear it with equanimity or tear it to shreds as reason dictates. We grow up in awareness of it and register its appearances forever after: on the sporting hero and the venal politician, on the captain of industry and the weekend cricket player, and every year under a dismal November sky, on men who are young, old, or unbelievably ancient at the Armistice Day parade.

P.L. Sells & Co. Ltd. has been making regimental ties for fifty years, and we are the only British firm left—a tiny business employing fifteen people—that offers a comprehensive, off-the-shelf service to the regiments, tailors, and old-fashioned men's outfitters who are our customers. An order received before 4 o'clock in the afternoon for any of the four hundred or so designs that we stock will be delivered early the next morning, courtesy of the Royal Mail, whose service we never tire of criticizing.

This book is a complete photographic record of our 1998 catalog. You will find here the designs of all the British military ties for which there is still a demand, together with those of the major public schools, universities, and Oxford colleges.

Our catalog has evolved over the years, particularly in the army section as old regiments have been merged into new ones, and these in their turn have disappeared in further amalgamations. The regular army of 1945, however, is still represented almost in its entirety.

With each year that passes our sales of regimental ties decrease. When the stock card shows that a design is selling at a rate of less than one a year, we discuss whether it is time to discontinue it. And we hesitate, knowing that as soon as we do, there will be calls from all over the country as the grandchildren of some last survivor go from shop to shop in search of this precious, potent symbol.

How much longer will it all last? When will the significant tie become really obsolete? I can only report that there is no sign yet. We are putting new designs into make every week, and they all seem to have a staying power that goes beyond every expectation. The oldest seem to be maintained by age itself. The Indian Army Association has ordered its ties from us for as long as I have worked in the business, three dozen a year, regular as clockwork. Colonel Emerson's letters used to be slightly apologetic: "Such a small order I'm afraid, there are not many of us left." Most recently he reports, "We still need more, my old boys are refusing to die off."

— *Christopher Sells*

P.L. Sells & Co. Ltd.
6/7 Stapleton House
110 Clifton Street
London EC2A 4HT

Royal Armoured Corps—Cavalry

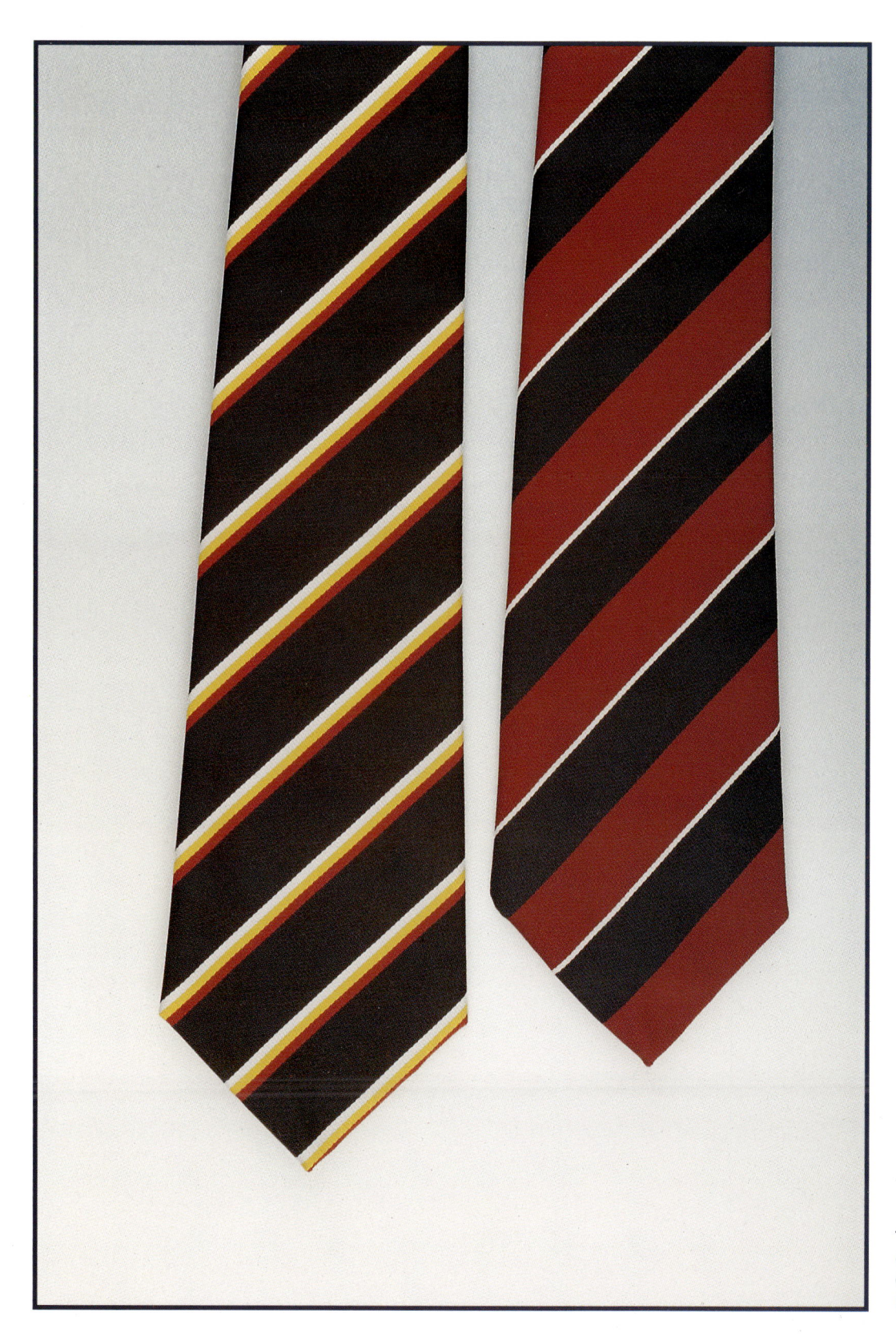

The Royal Scots Dragoon Guards (Carabiniers & Greys); 1st The Queen's Dragoon Guards

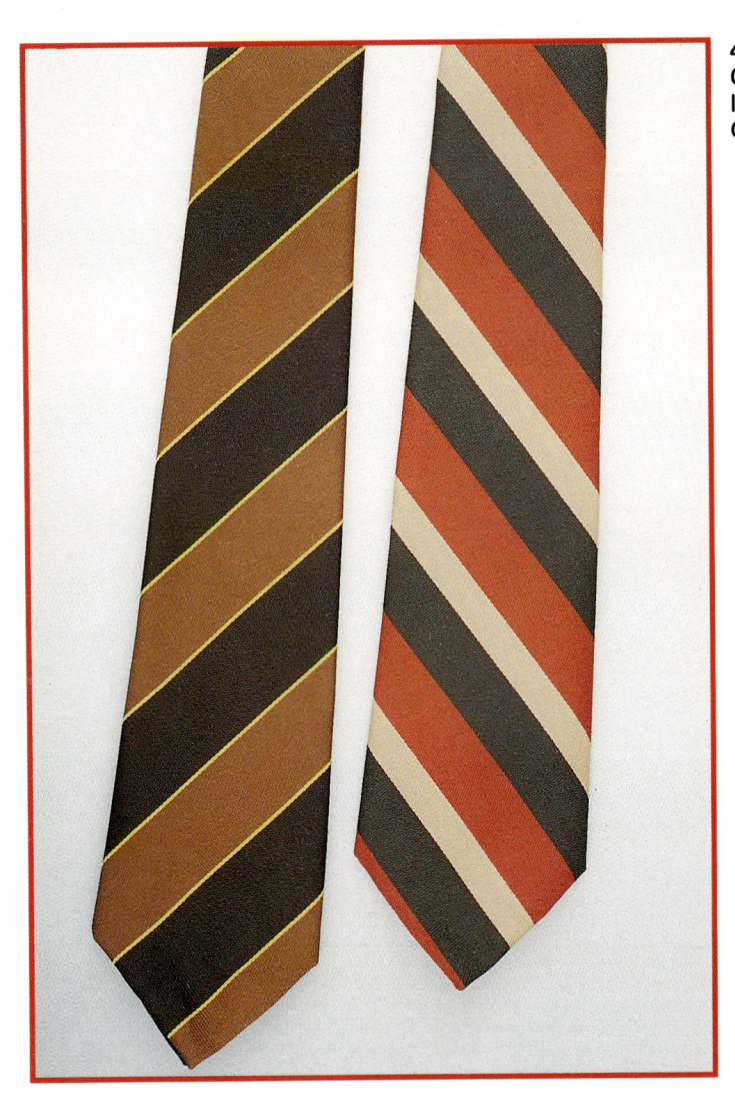

4th/7th Royal Dragoon Guards; 5th Royal Inniskilling Dragoon Guards

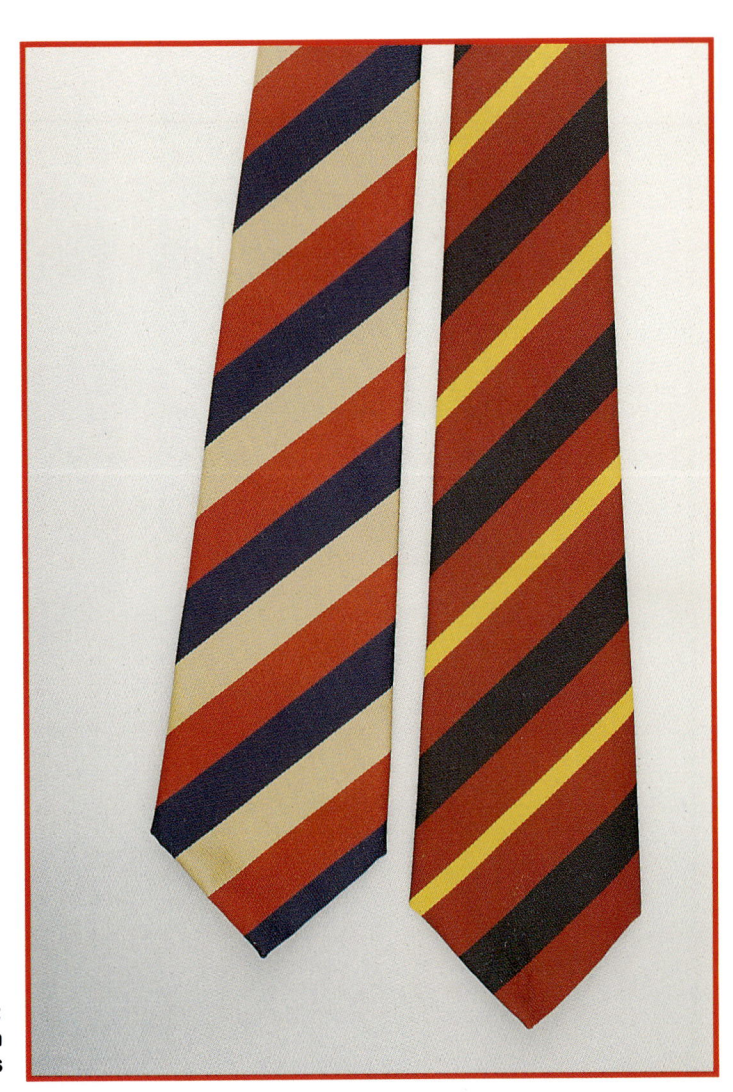

The Light Dragoons; 1st King's Dragoon Guards

6

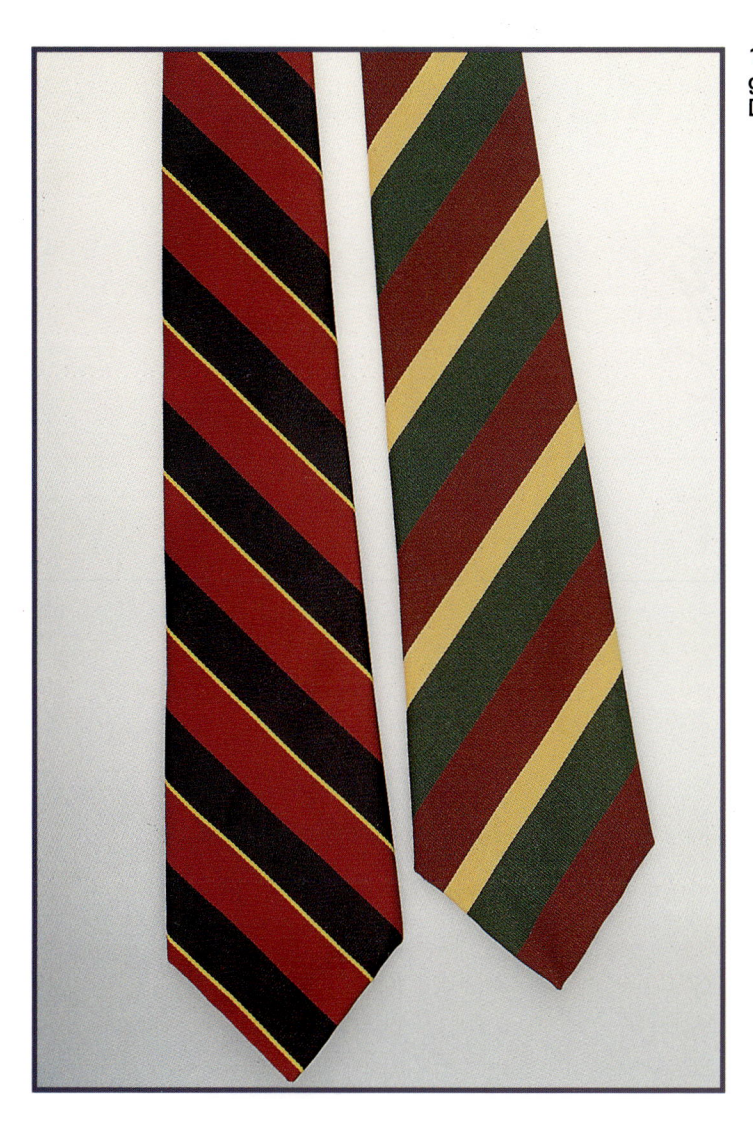

1st The Royal Dragoons; The Royal Dragoon Guards

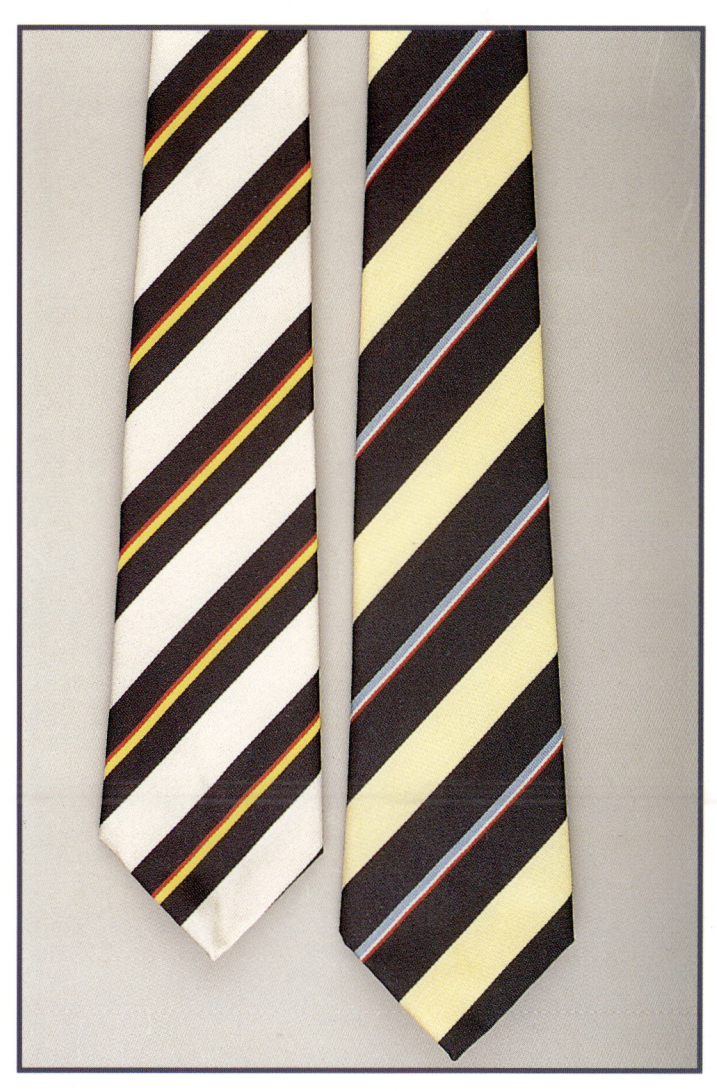

The Royal Scots Greys (2nd Dragoons); The Queen's Own Hussars (3rd/7th)

7

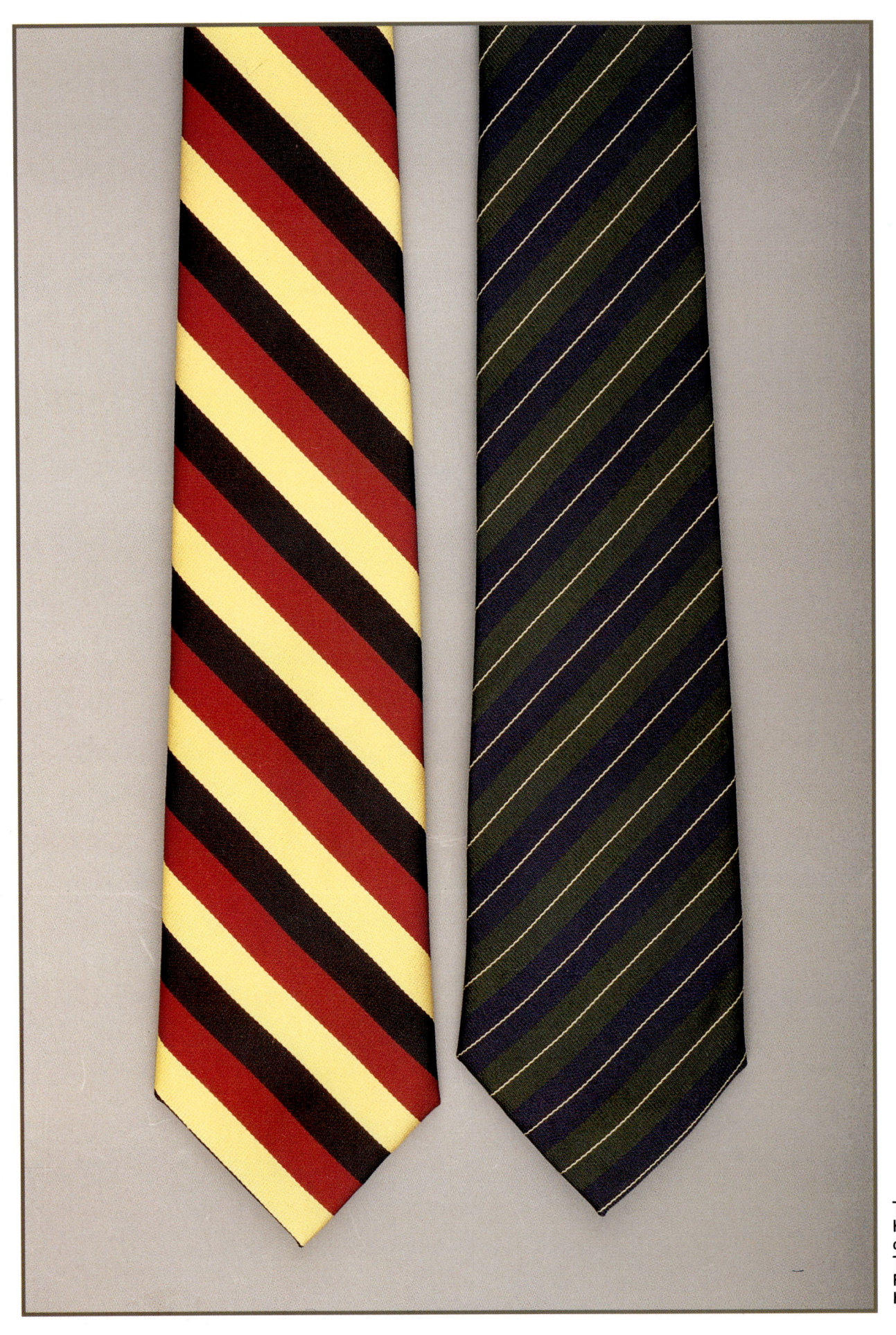

The Royal
Hussars (Prince
of Wales's Own);
The Queen's
Royal Irish
Hussars

14th/20th King's Hussars; 13th/18th Royal Hussars (Queen Mary's Own)

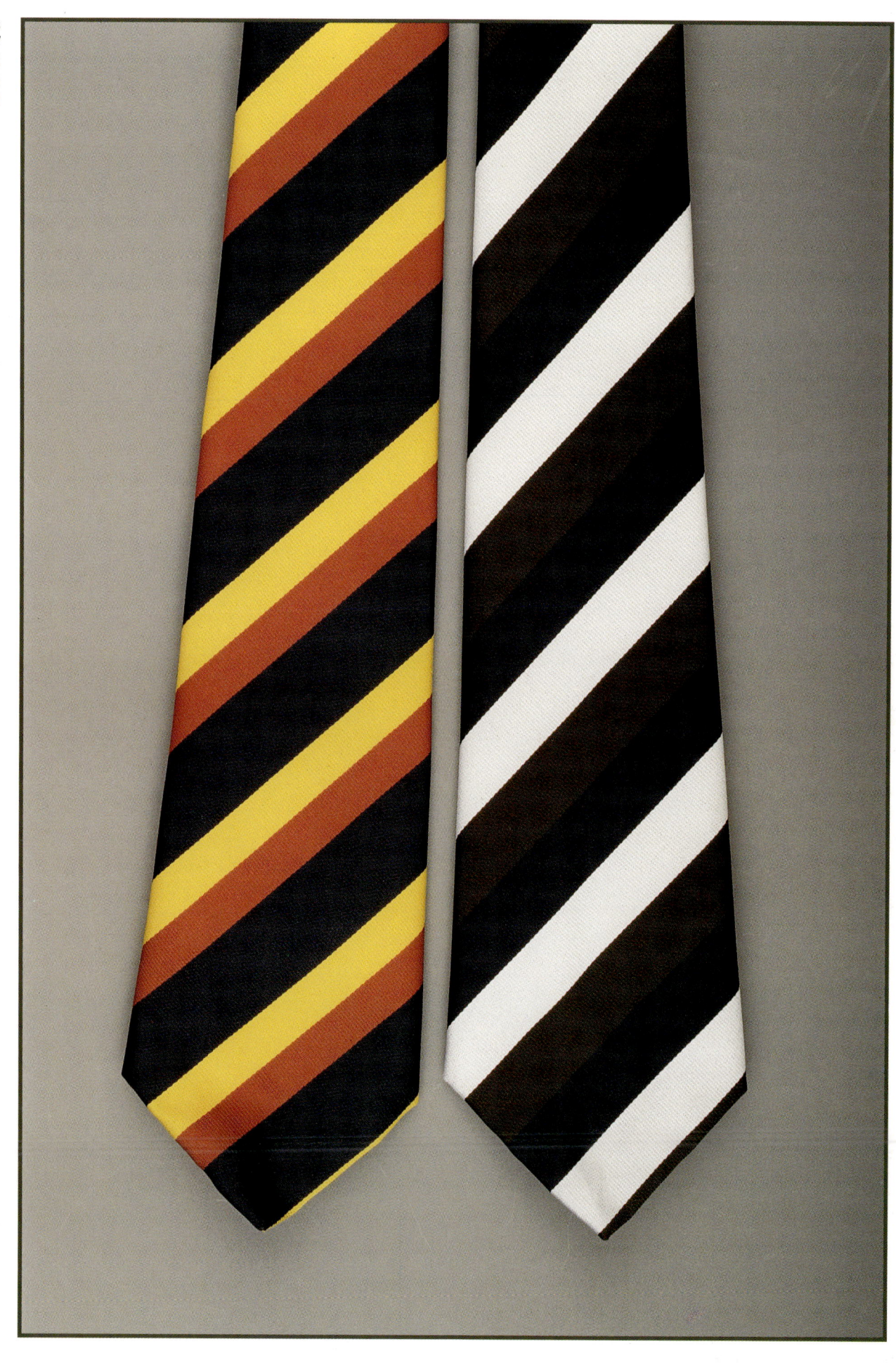

3rd The King's Own Hussars (old pattern); 15th/19th The King's Royal Hussars

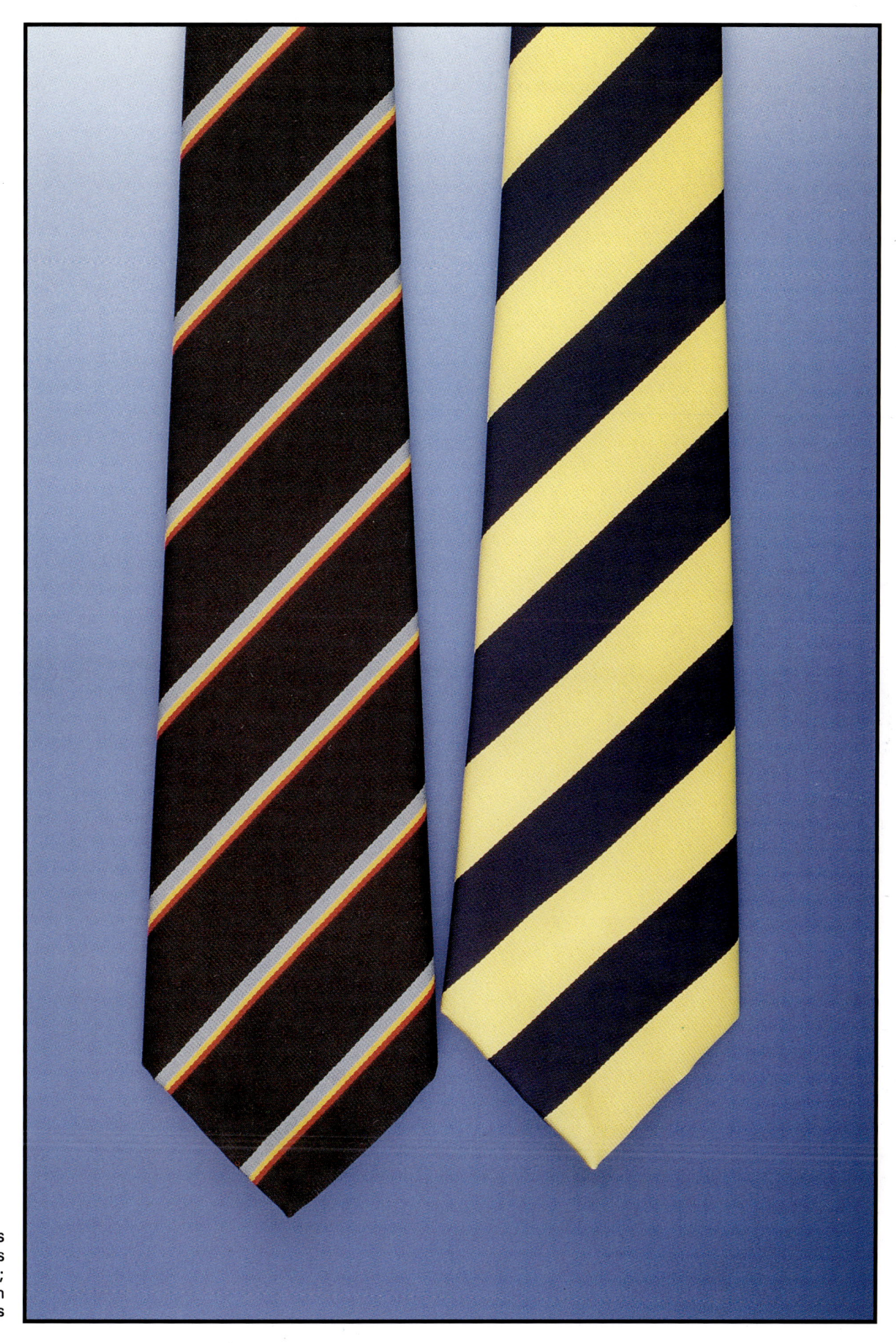

3rd The King's
Own Hussars
(new pattern);
4th Queen's Own
Hussars

11th Hussars (Prince Albert's own); 10th Royal Hussars (Prince of Wales's Own)

8th King's Royal Irish Hussars; 7th Queen's Own Hussars

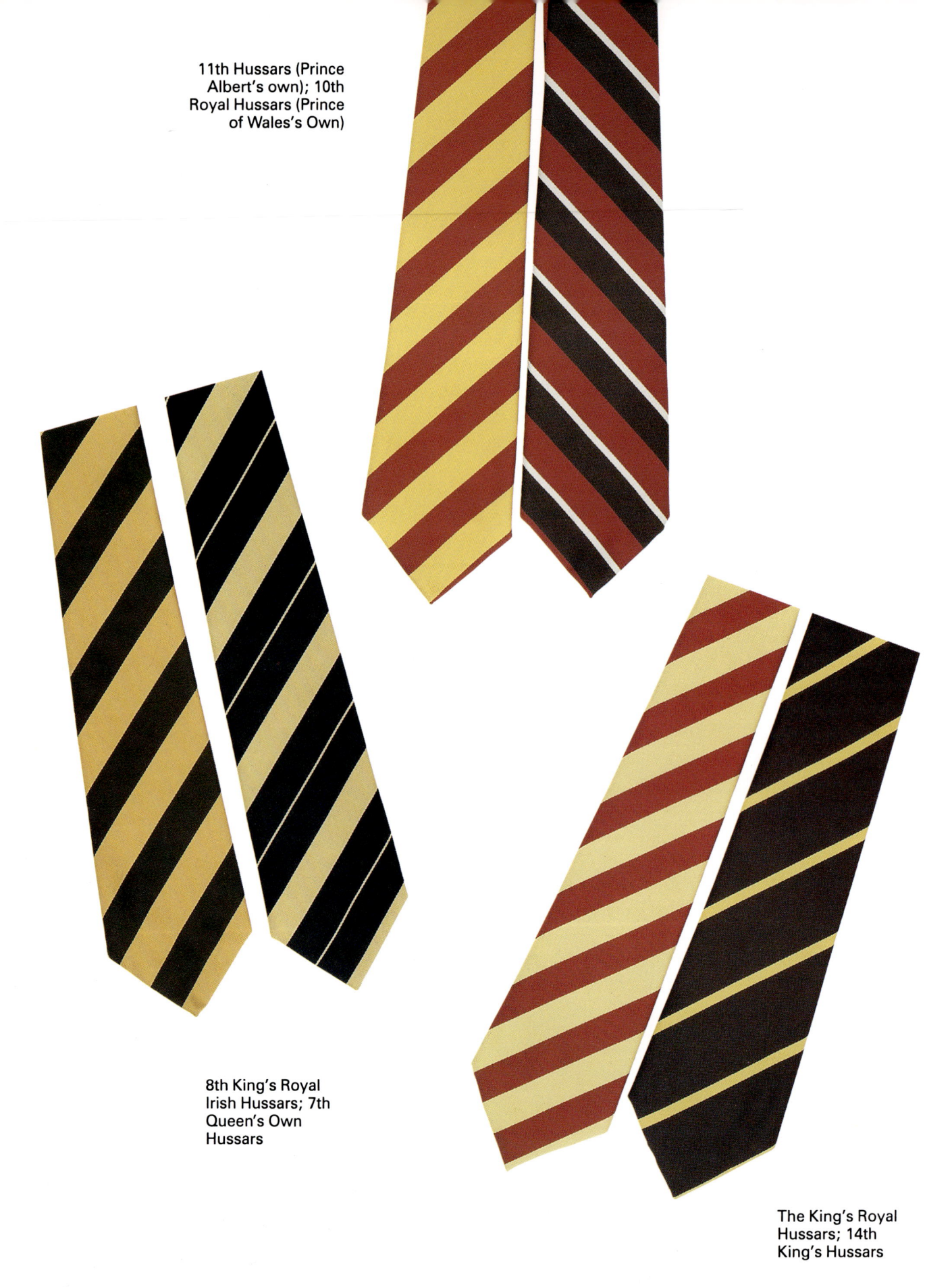

The King's Royal Hussars; 14th King's Hussars

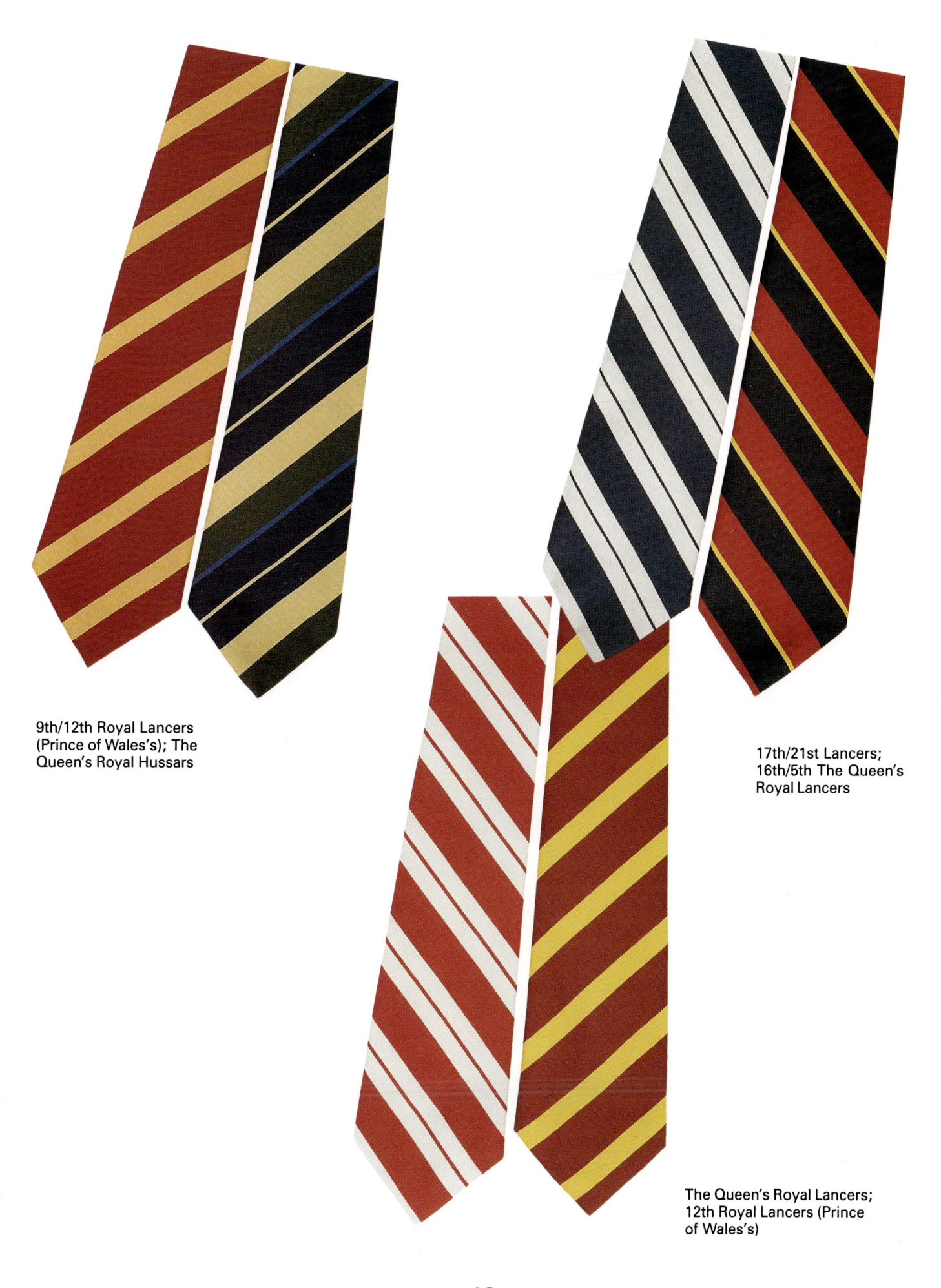

9th/12th Royal Lancers
(Prince of Wales's); The
Queen's Royal Hussars

17th/21st Lancers;
16th/5th The Queen's
Royal Lancers

The Queen's Royal Lancers;
12th Royal Lancers (Prince
of Wales's)

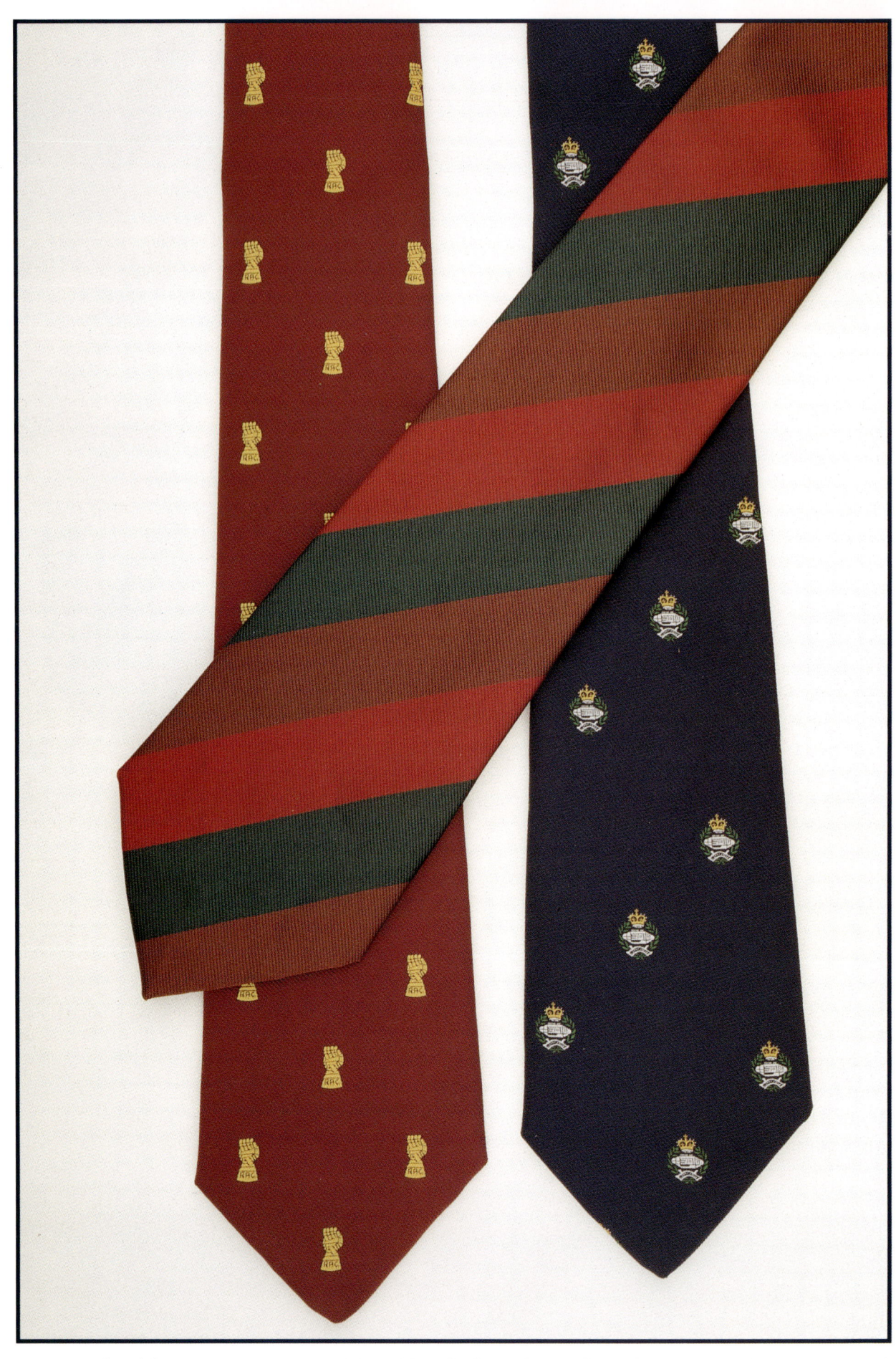

Royal Armoured Corps (maroon); Royal Tank Regiment (crest); Royal Tank Regiment (stripe)

Regiments and Yeomanry

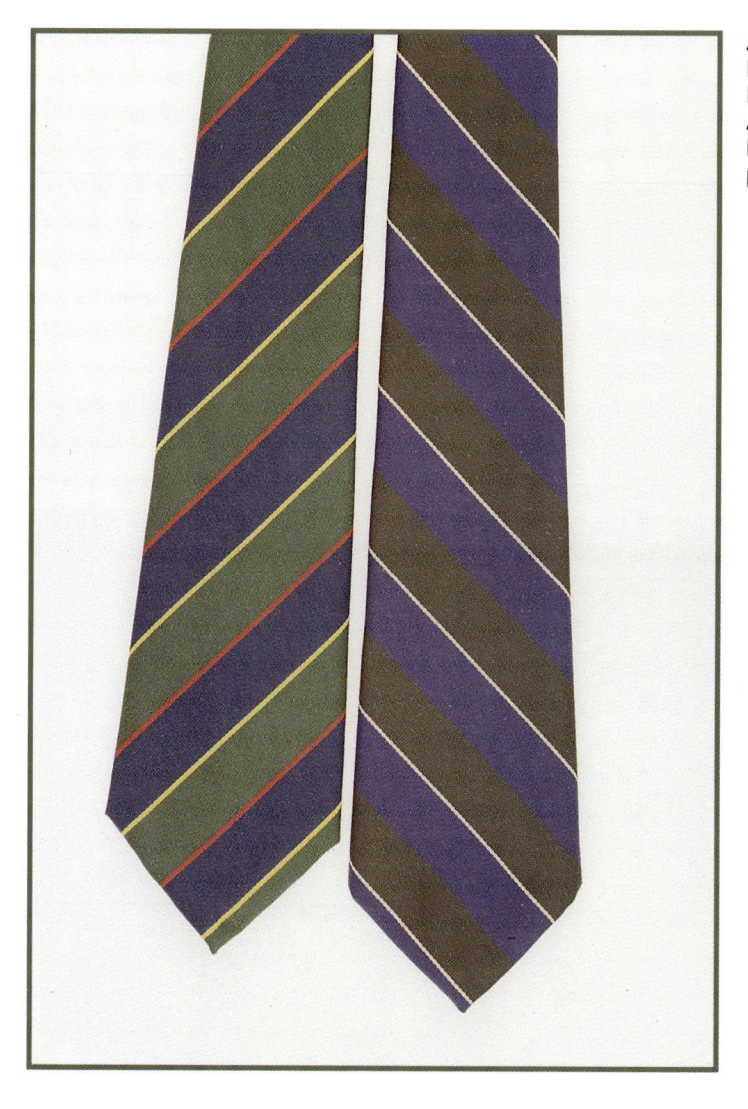

Argyll & Sutherland Highlanders (Princess Louise's, 1st Batt.); Argyll & Sutherland Highlanders (new pattern)

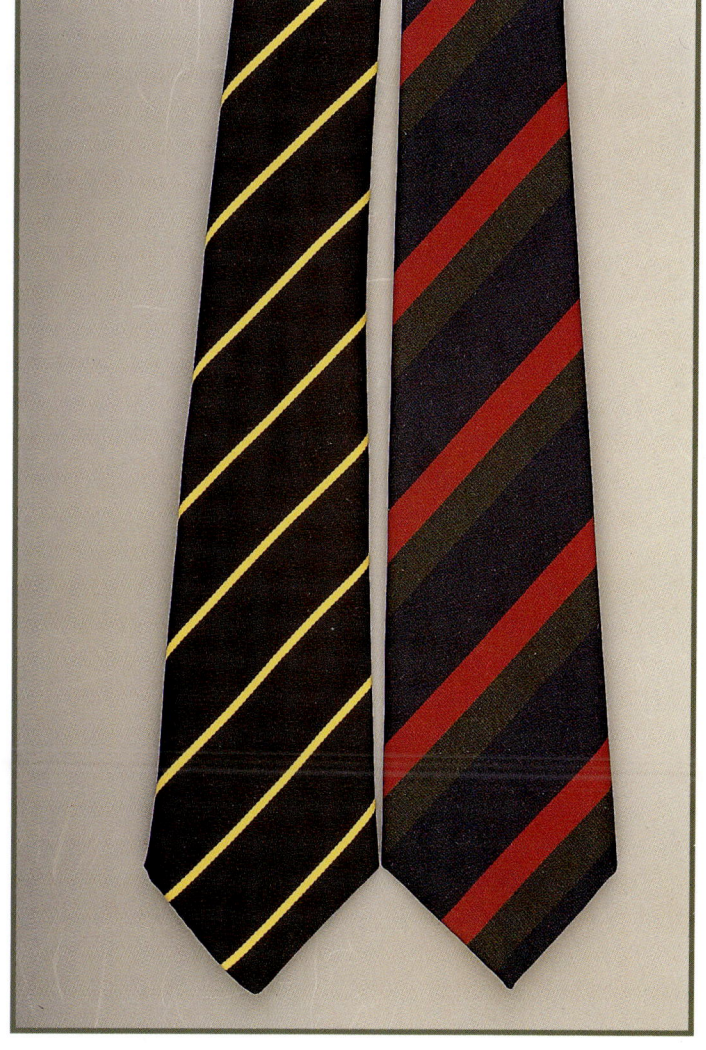

Bedfordshire & Hertfordshire Regiment; Black Watch (Royal Highland Regiment)

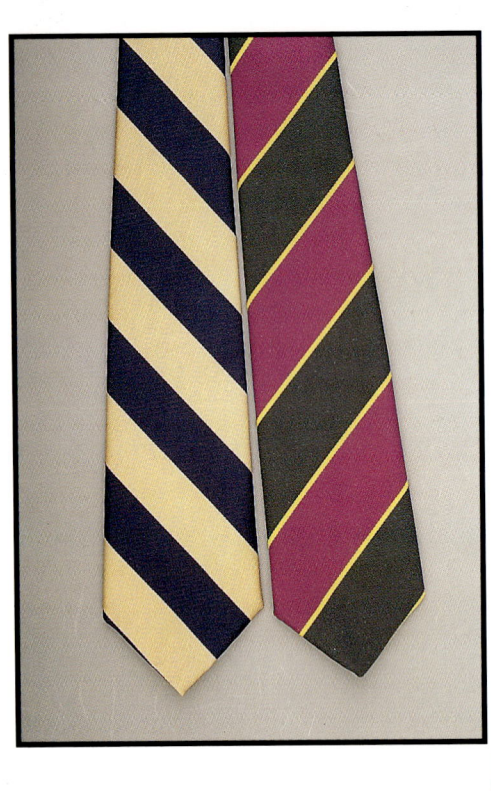

The Buffs (Royal East Kent Regiment); Border Regiment

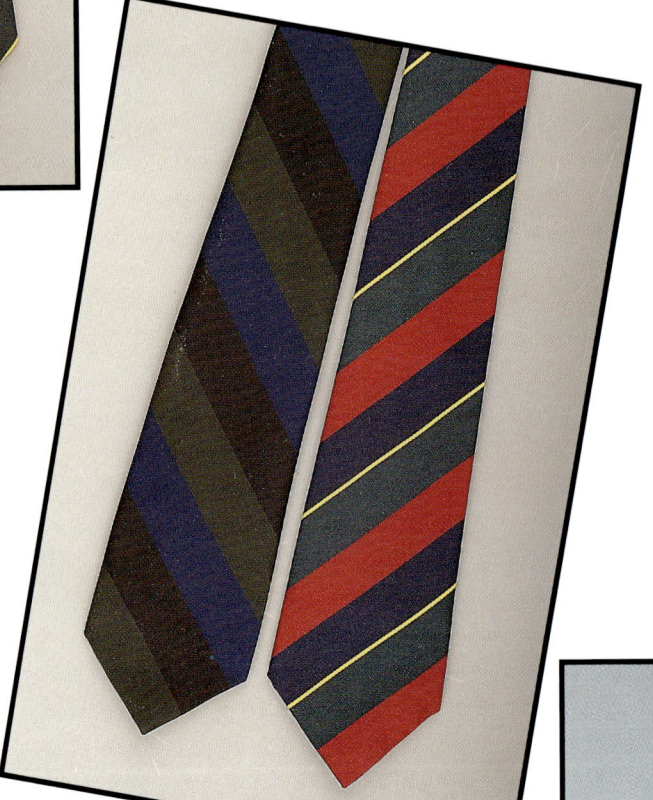

Cameronians (Scottish Rifles); Cameron Highlanders, The Queen's Own

Cheshire Regiment; Coldstream Guards

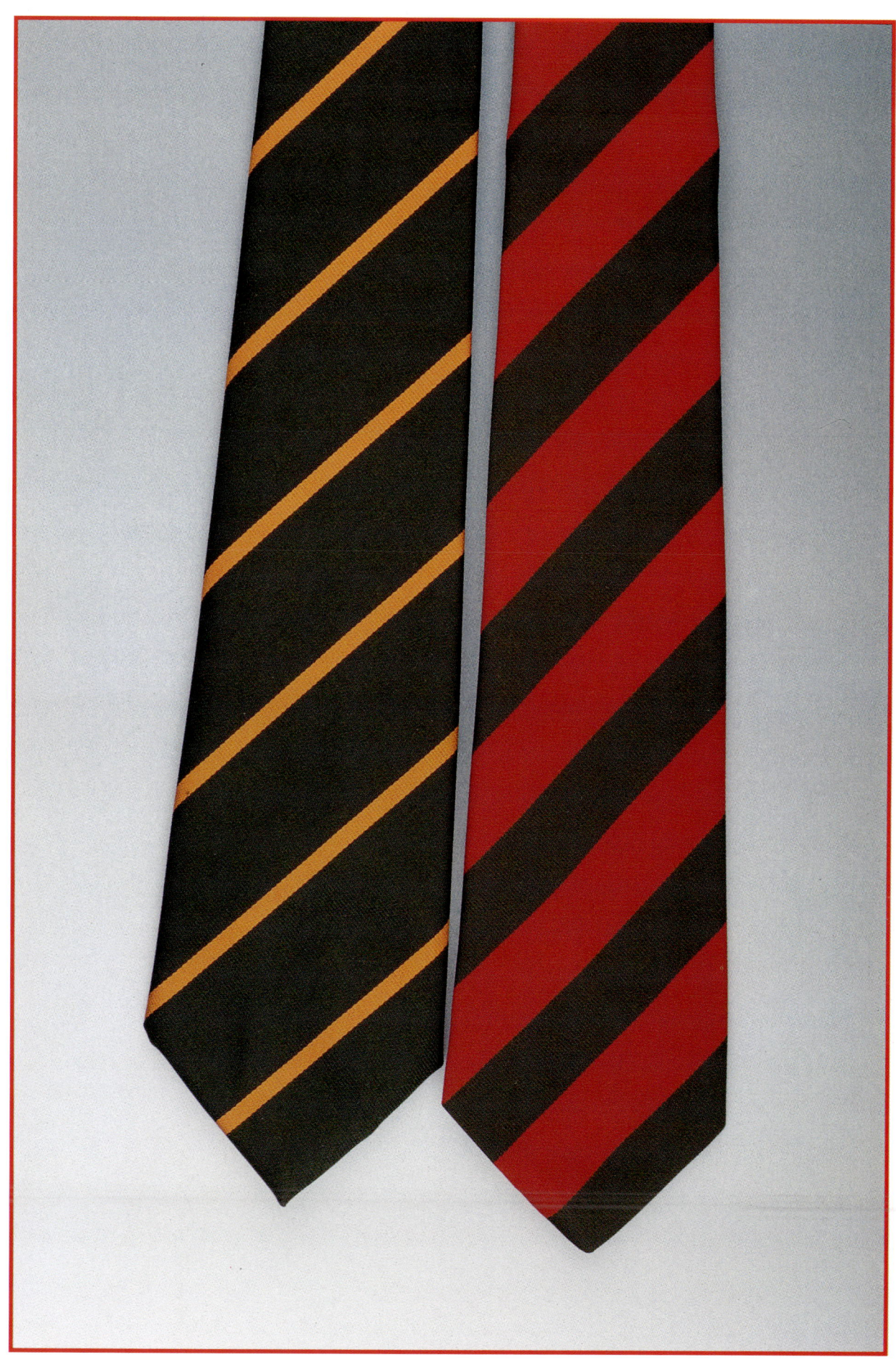

Devonshire and Dorset Regiment; Devonshire Regiment

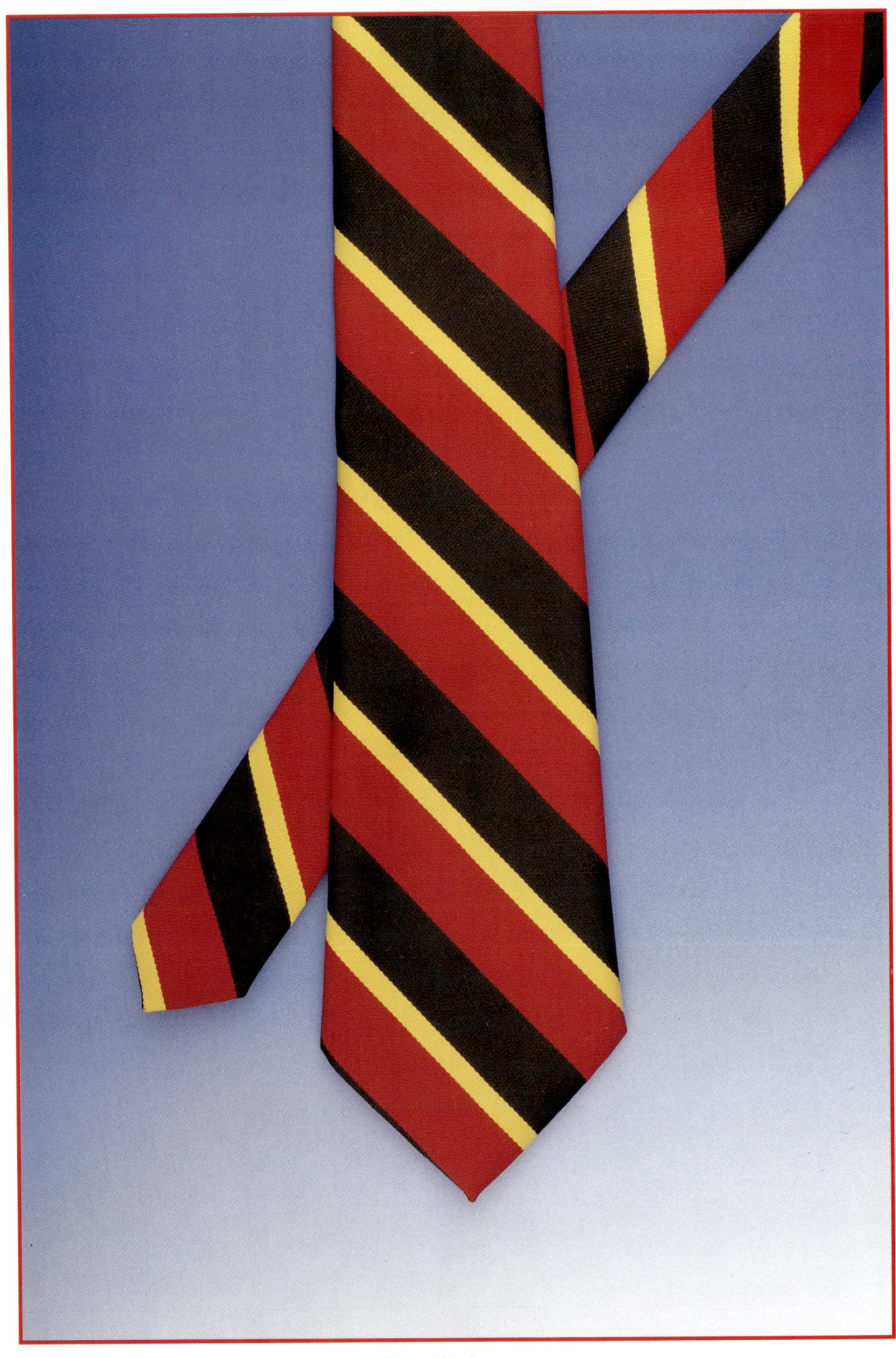

Dorset Regiment

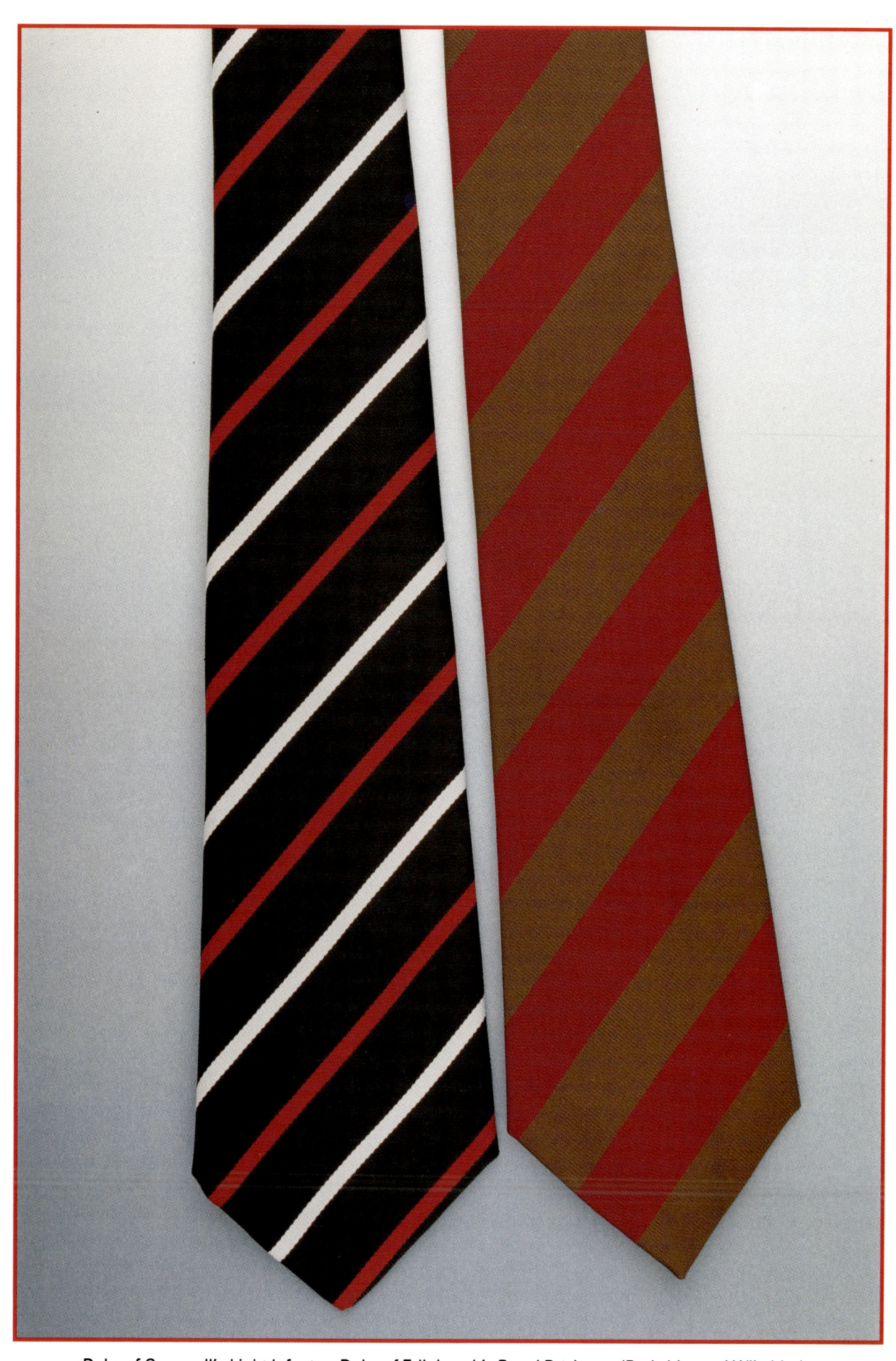

Duke of Cornwall's Light Infantry; Duke of Edinburgh's Royal Regiment (Berkshire and Wiltshire)

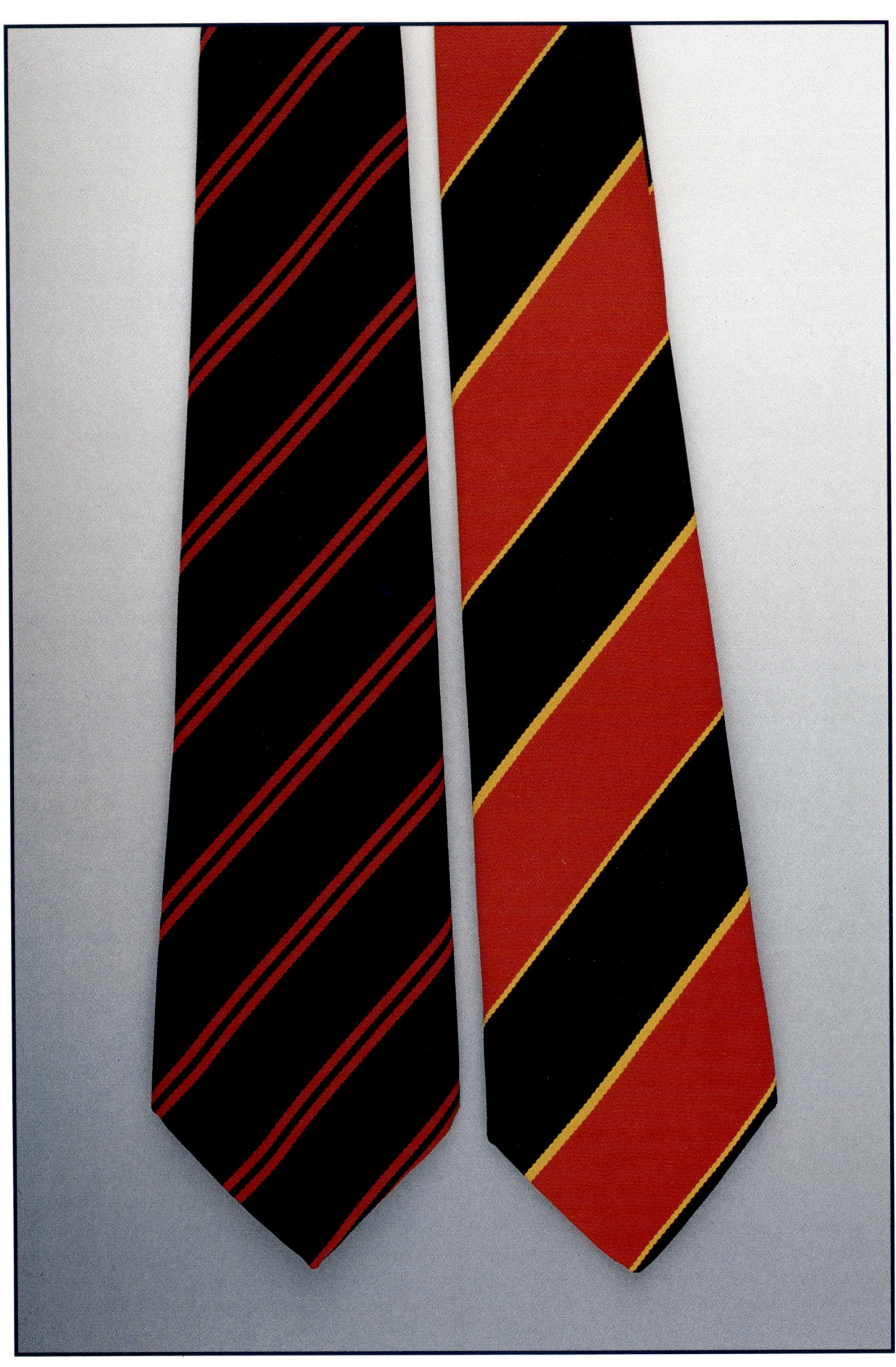

Duke of Edinburgh's Royal Regiment; Duke of Lancaster's Own Yeomanry

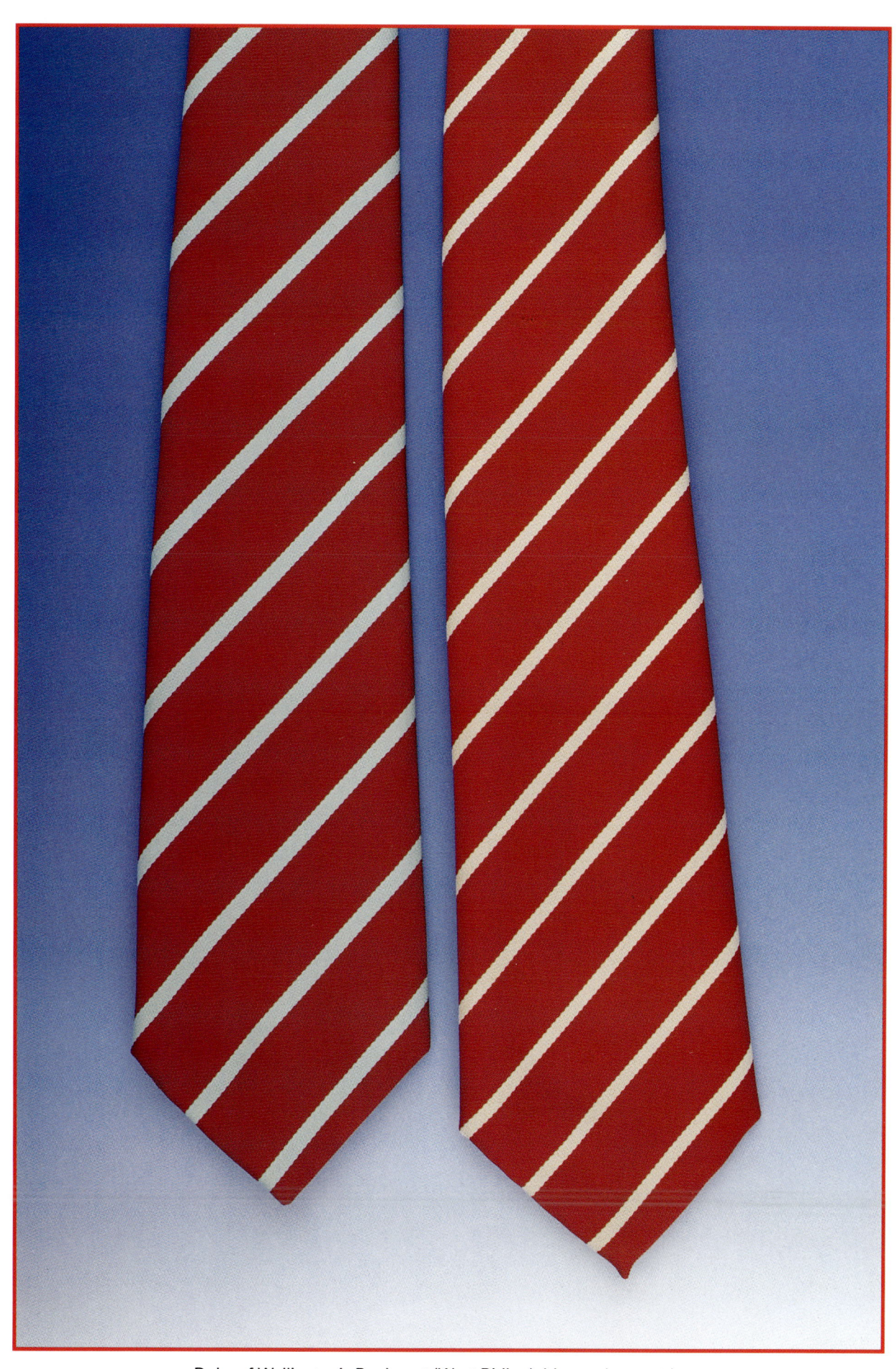

Duke of Wellington's Regiment (West Riding), blue and grey stripe

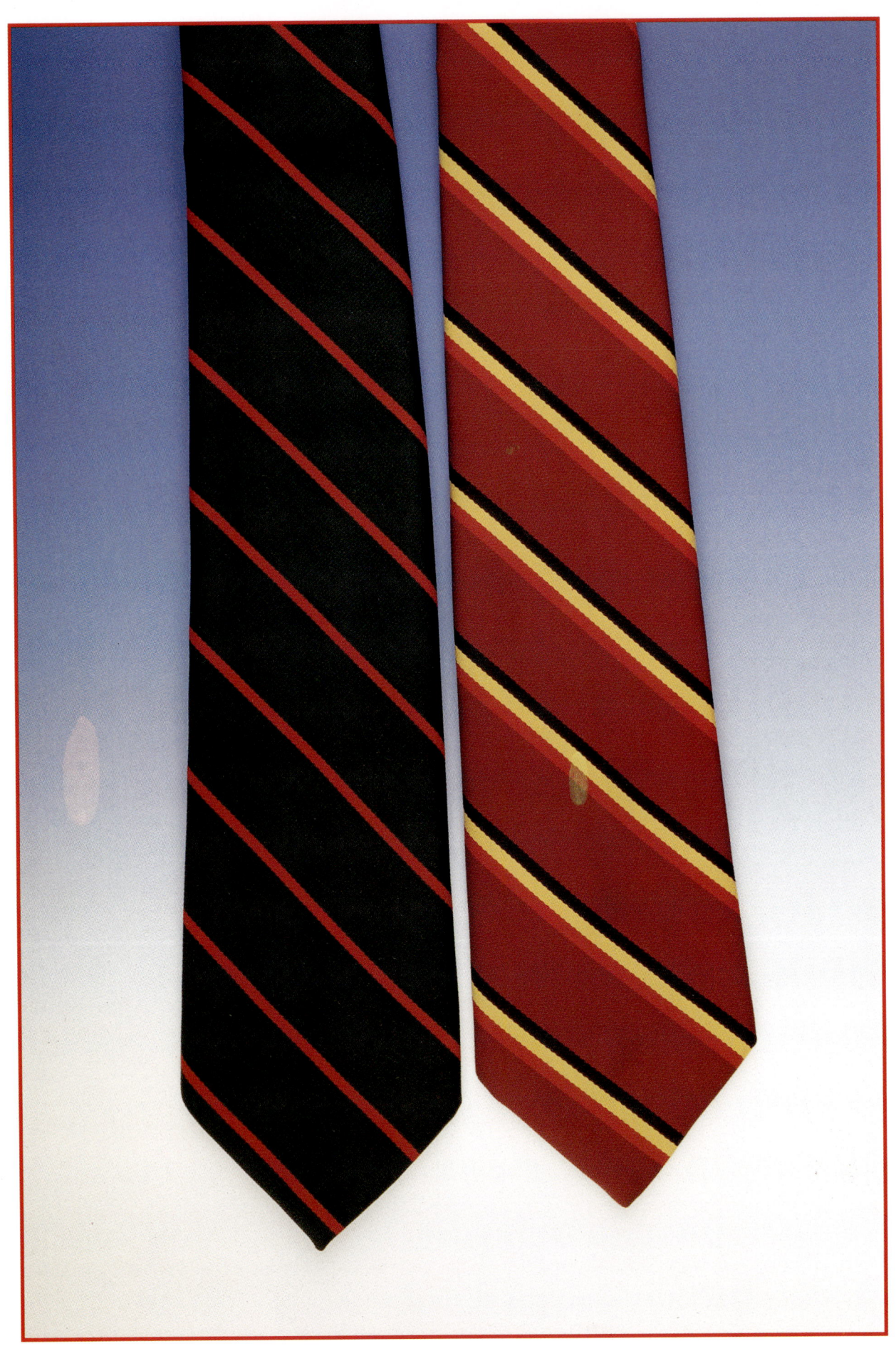

Durham Light Infantry; East Anglia Regiment

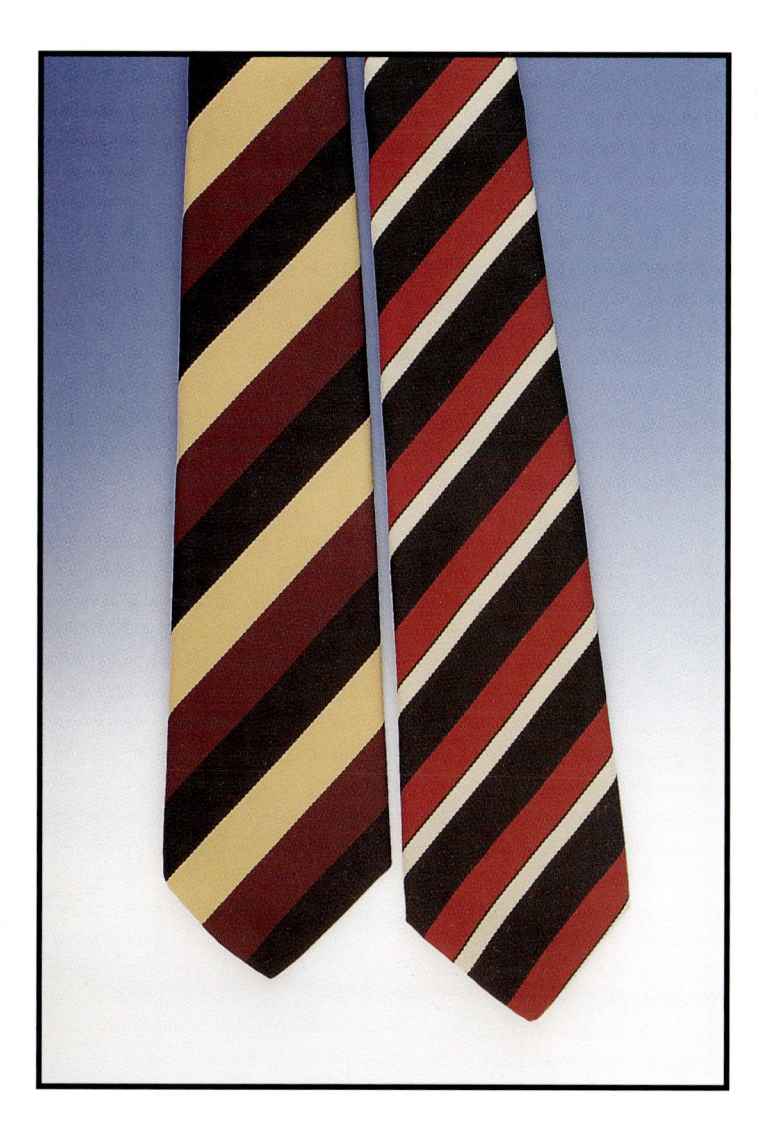

East Lancashire Regiment;
East Surrey Regiment

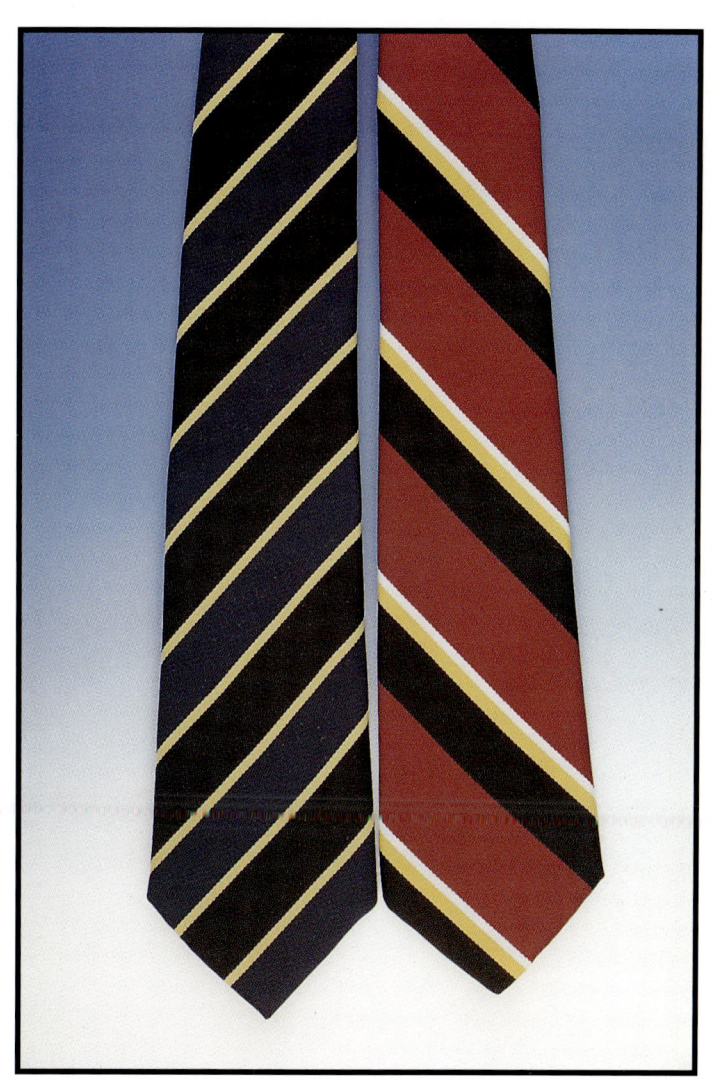

Essex Regiment; East
Yorkshire Regiment
(Duke of York's Own)

23

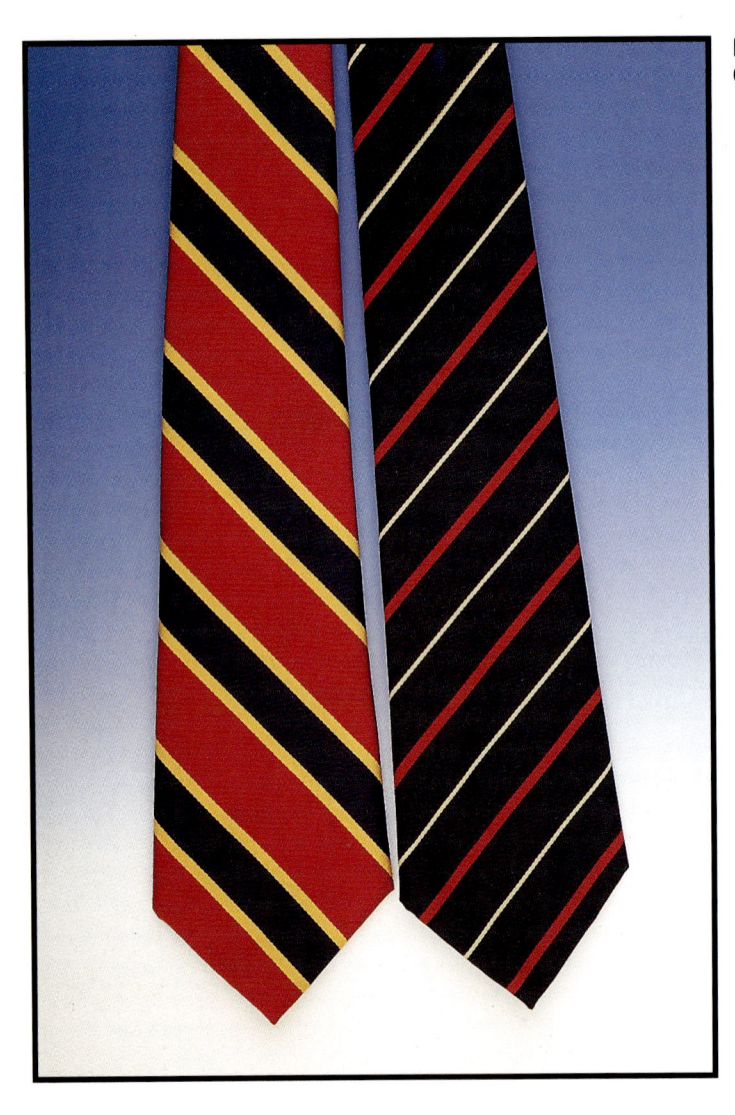

Fife and Forfar Yeomanry;
Gloucestershire Regiment

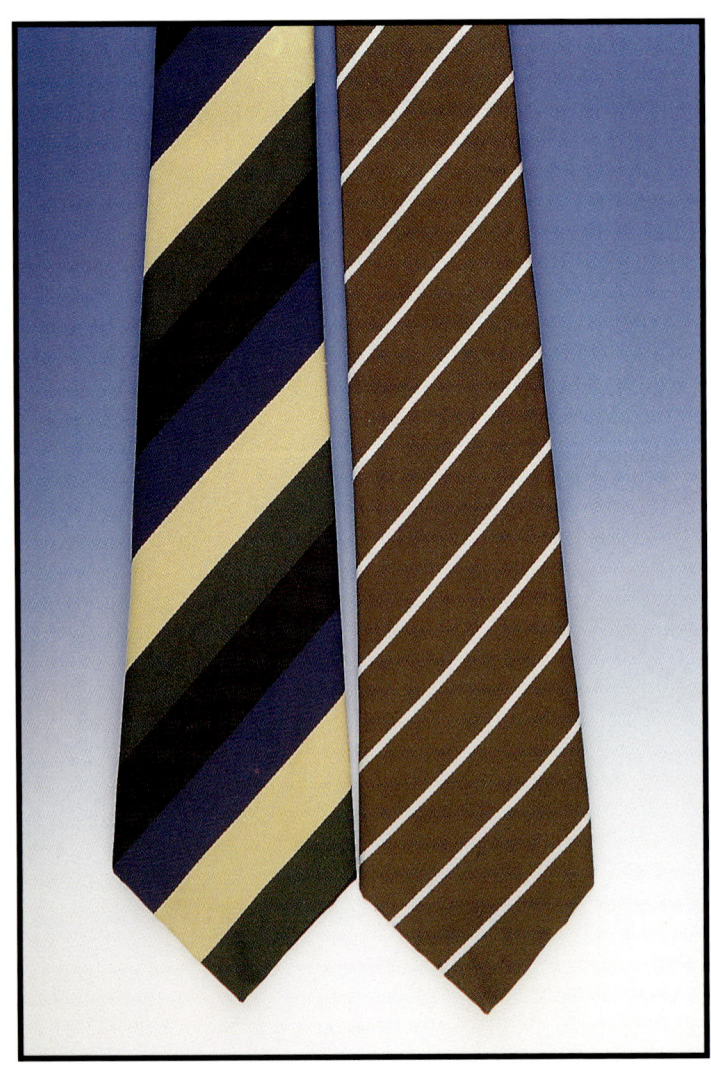

Gordon Highlanders;
Green Howards
(Alexandra, Princess of
Wales's Own Yorkshire
Regiment)

24

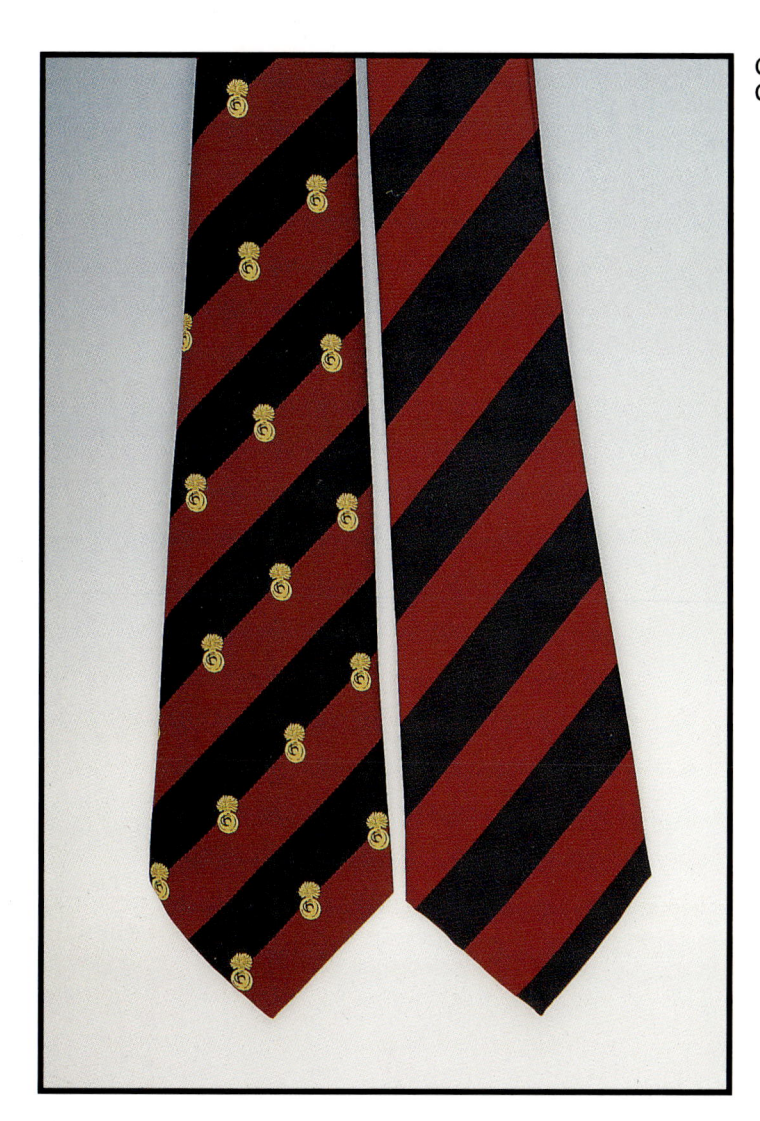

Grenadier Guards;
Guards Brigade

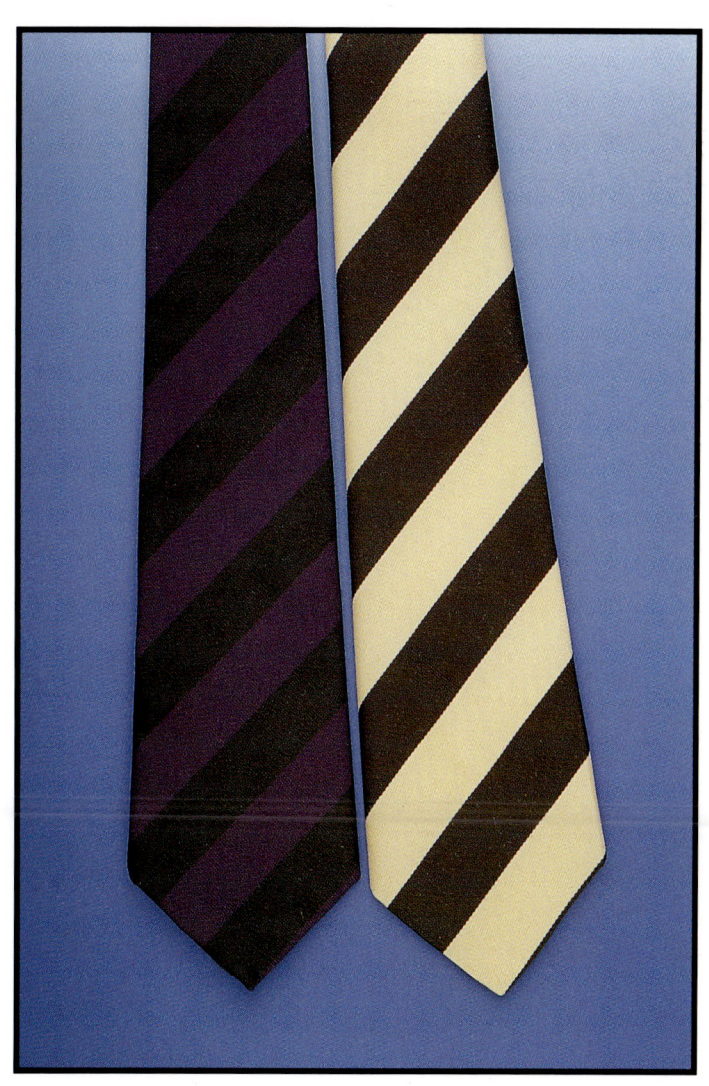

Highland Brigade;
Highland Light Infantry
(City of Glasgow
Regiment)

25

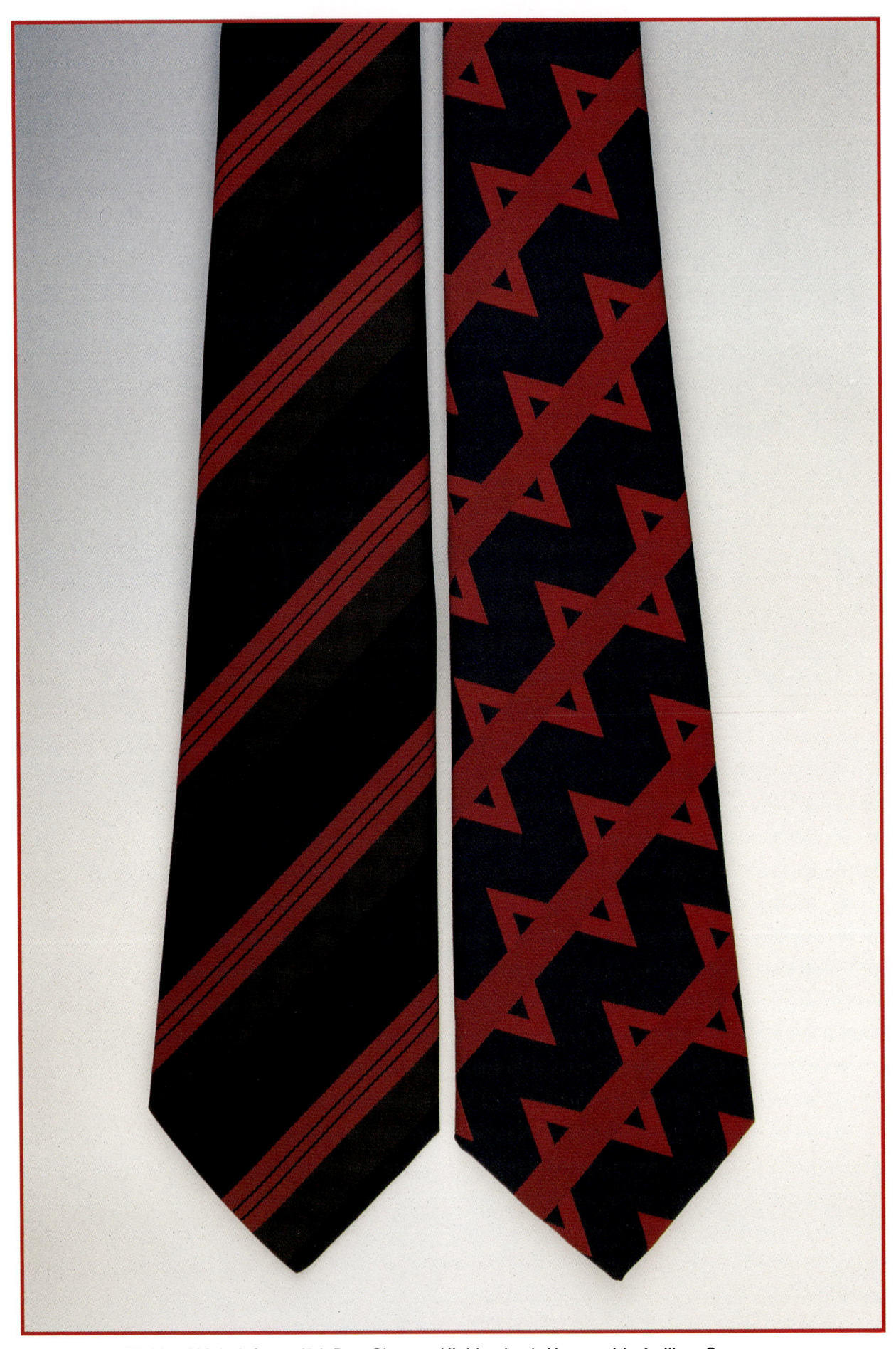

Highland Light Infantry (9th Batt. Glasgow Highlanders); Honourable Artillery Company

Inns of Court Regiment; Irish Guards

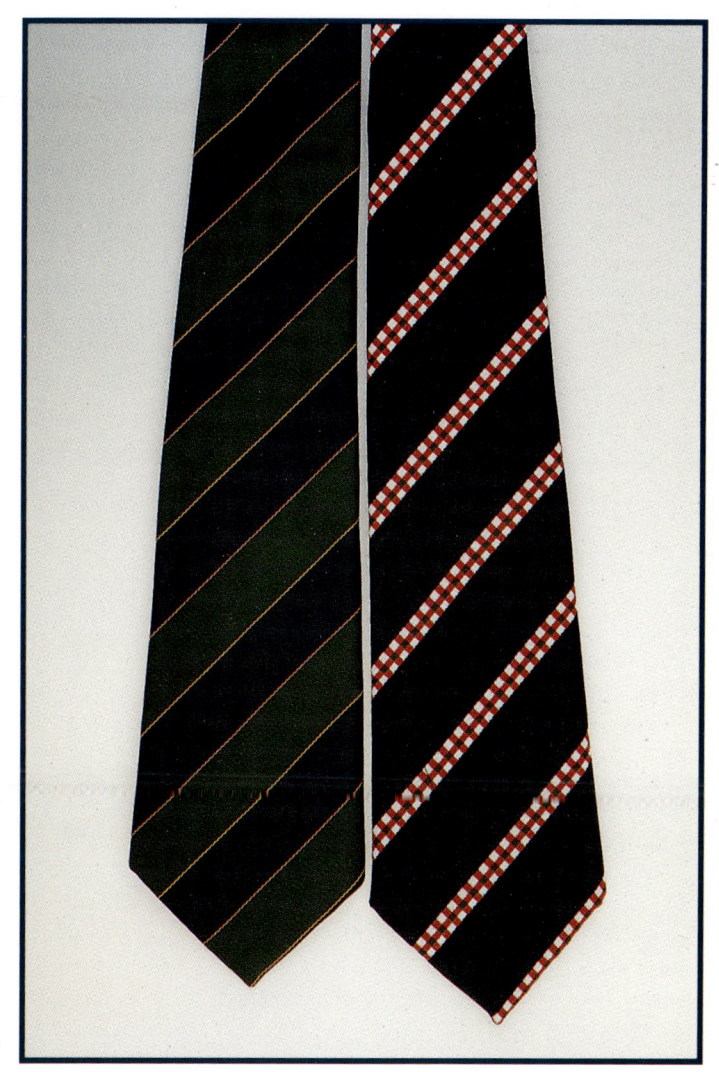

King's Own Royal Border Regiment; King's Own Scottish Borderers

27

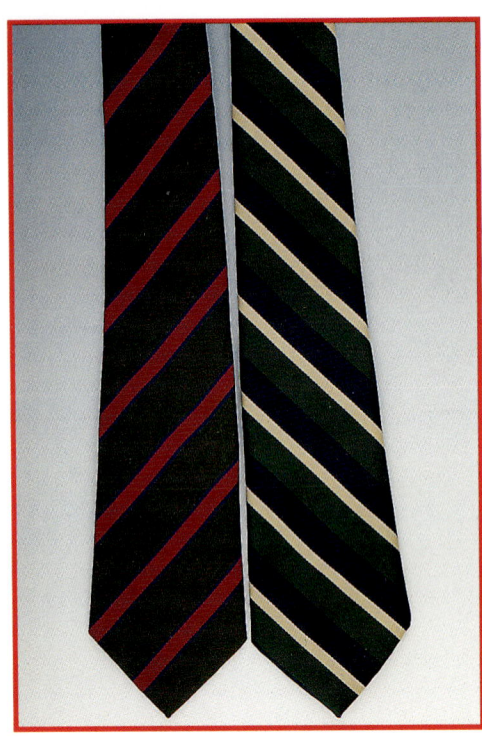

King's Regiment
(Manchester and
Liverpool); King's
Own Yorkshire
Light Infantry

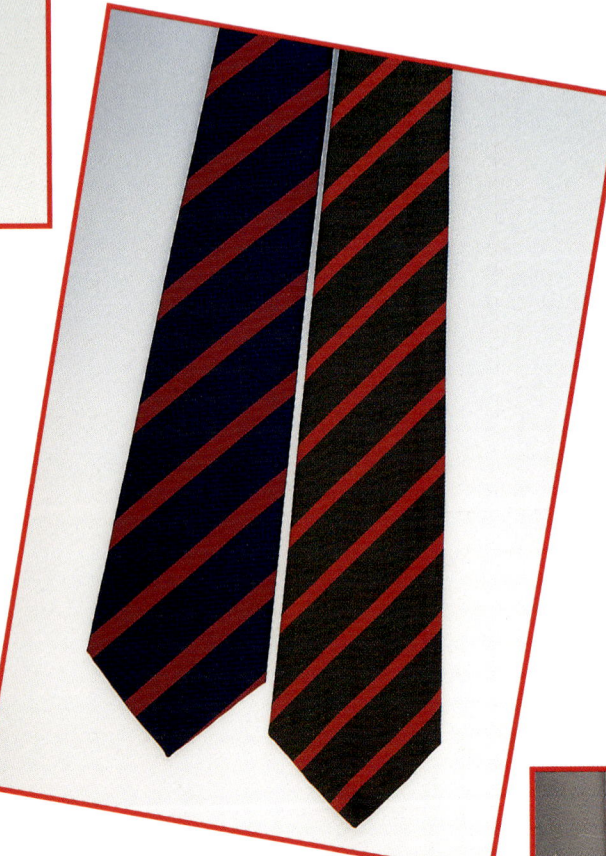

King's Regiment
(Liverpool); King's
Royal Rifle Corps

King's Shropshire
Light Infantry;
Lancashire Fusiliers

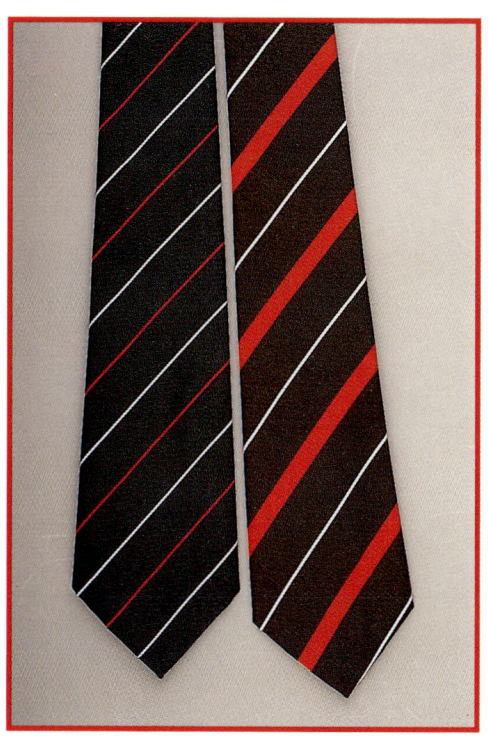

Light Infantry;
Light Infantry
(new 1995)

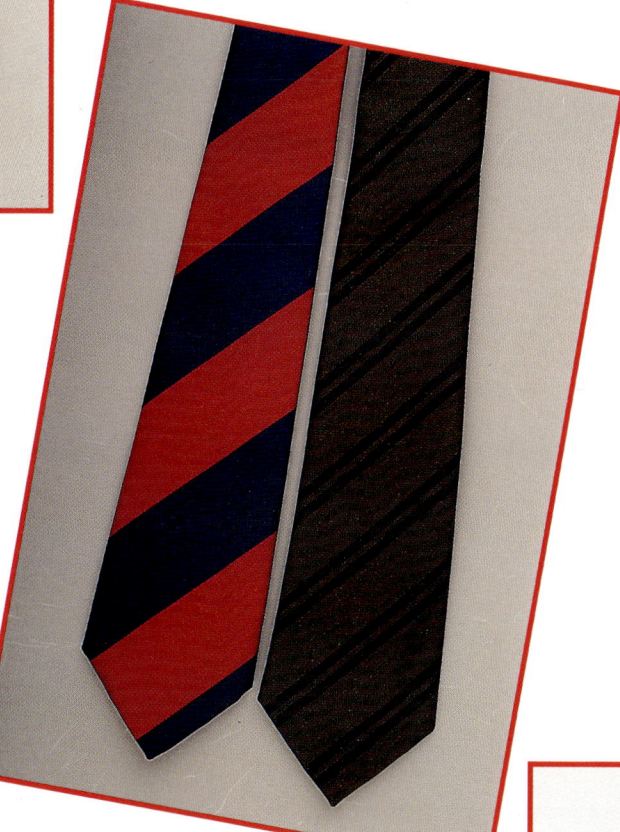

1st City of London
Regiment, Royal Fusiliers;
5th City of London
Regiment, London Rifle
Brigade

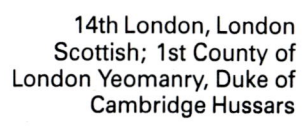

14th London, London
Scottish; 1st County of
London Yeomanry, Duke of
Cambridge Hussars

29

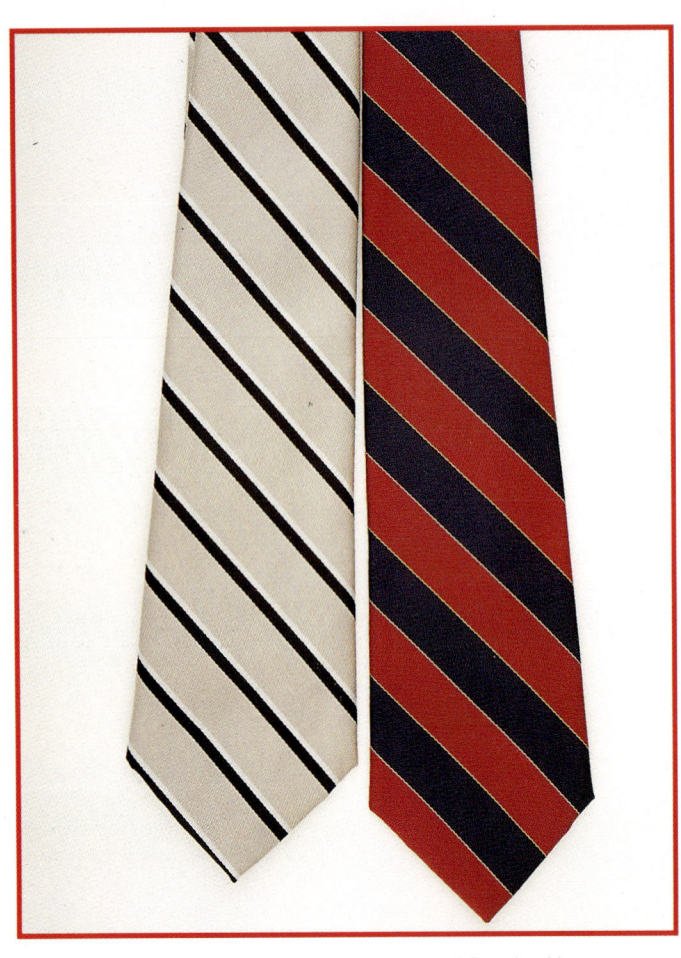

28th London, Artists' Rifles; Lothian and Border Horse

Middlesex Regiment (Duke of Cambridge's Own); Northamptonshire Regiment

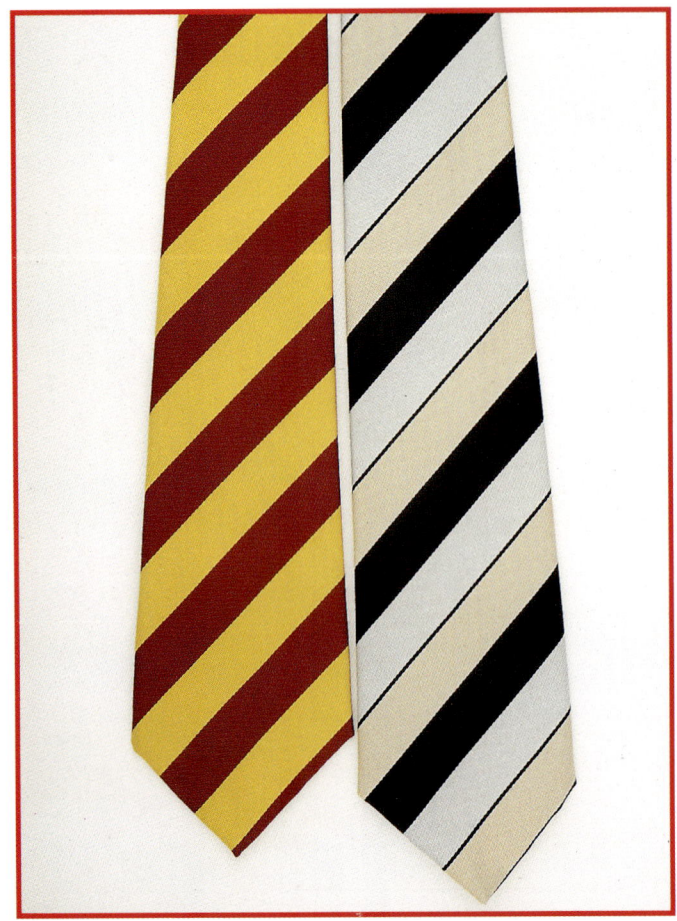

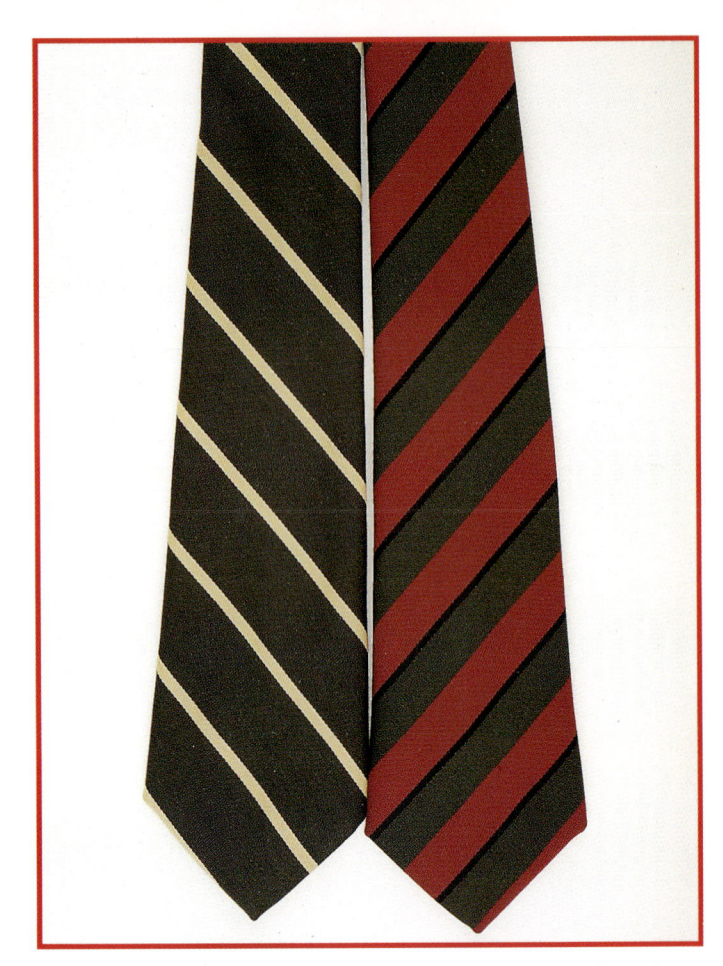

Manchester Regiment; Loyal Regiment (North Lancashire)

Northamptonshire Yeomanry; North Staffordshire Regiment (The Prince of Wales's)

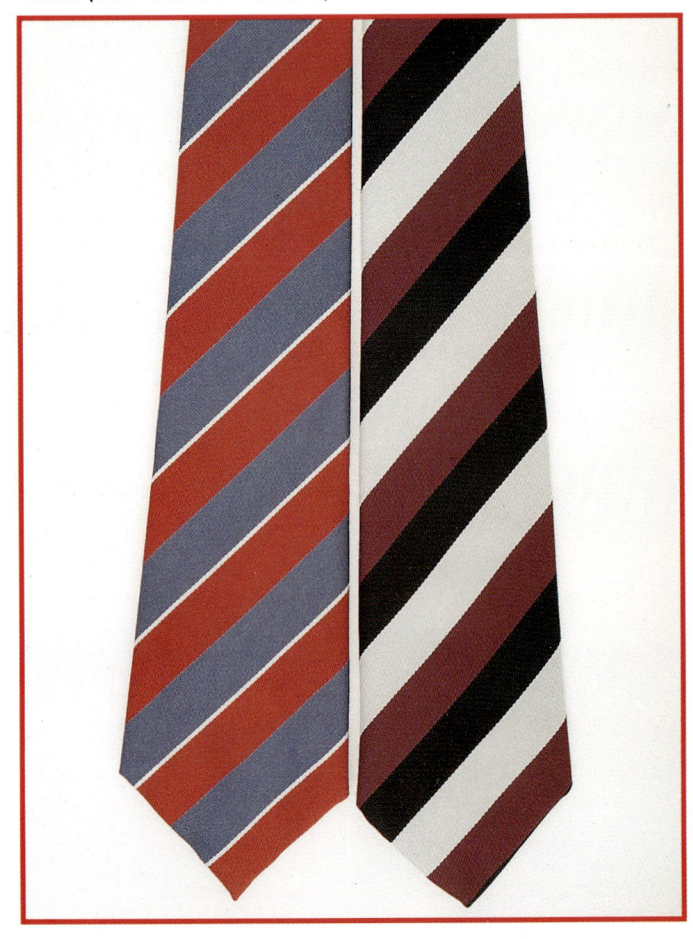

30

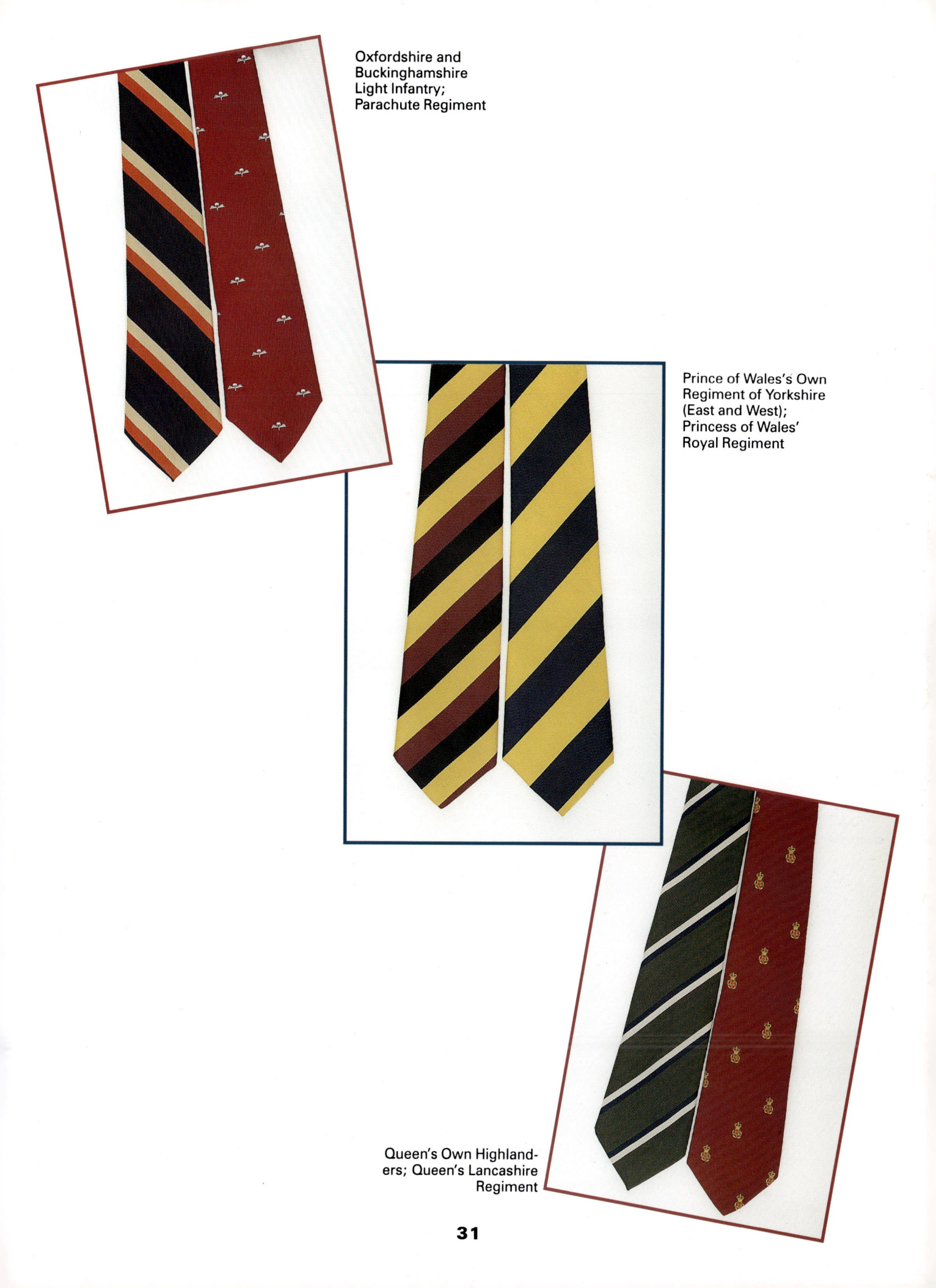

Oxfordshire and
Buckinghamshire
Light Infantry;
Parachute Regiment

Prince of Wales's Own
Regiment of Yorkshire
(East and West);
Princess of Wales'
Royal Regiment

Queen's Own Highlanders; Queen's Lancashire Regiment

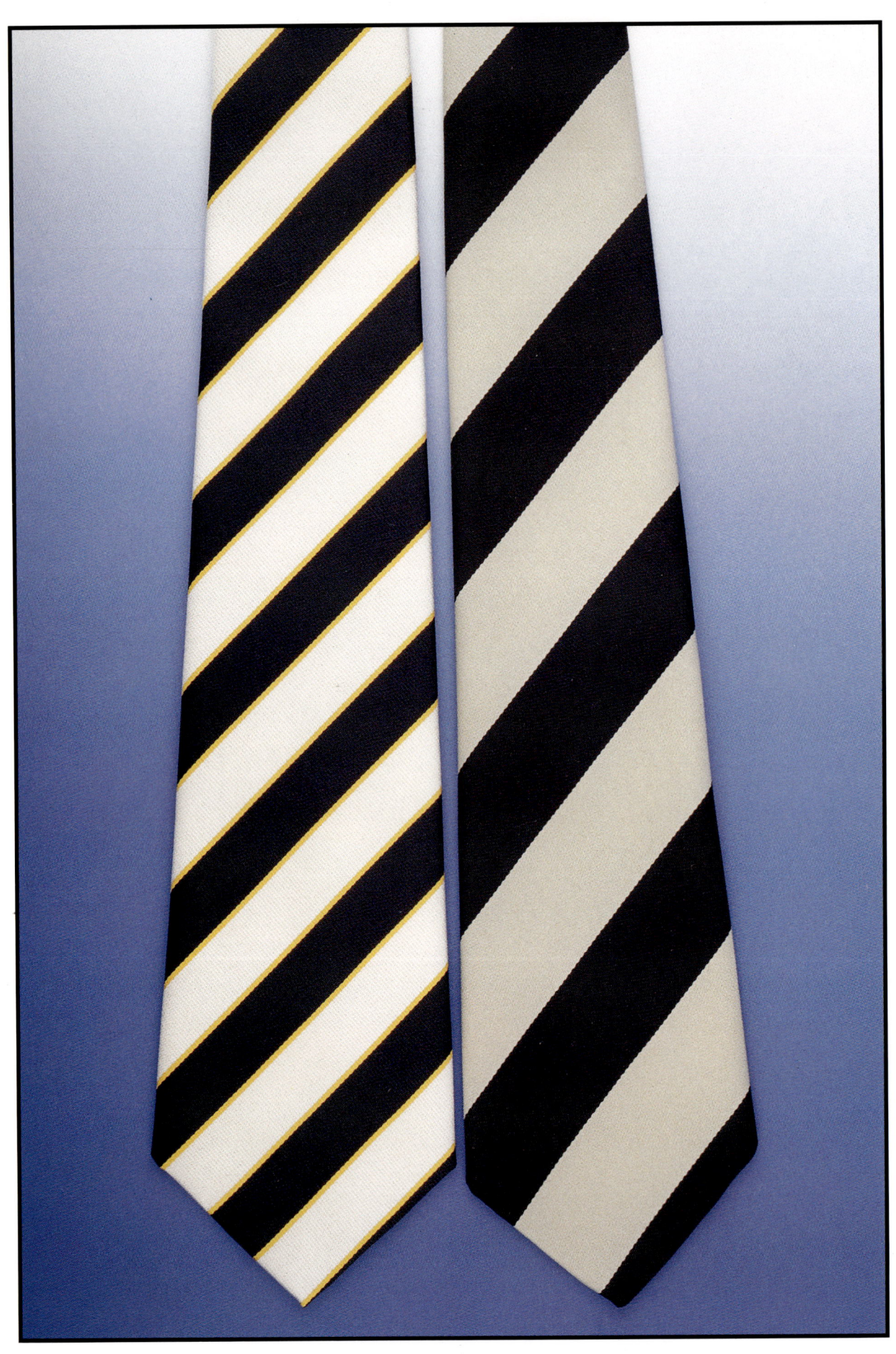

Queen's Regiment; Queen's Own Royal West Kent Regiment

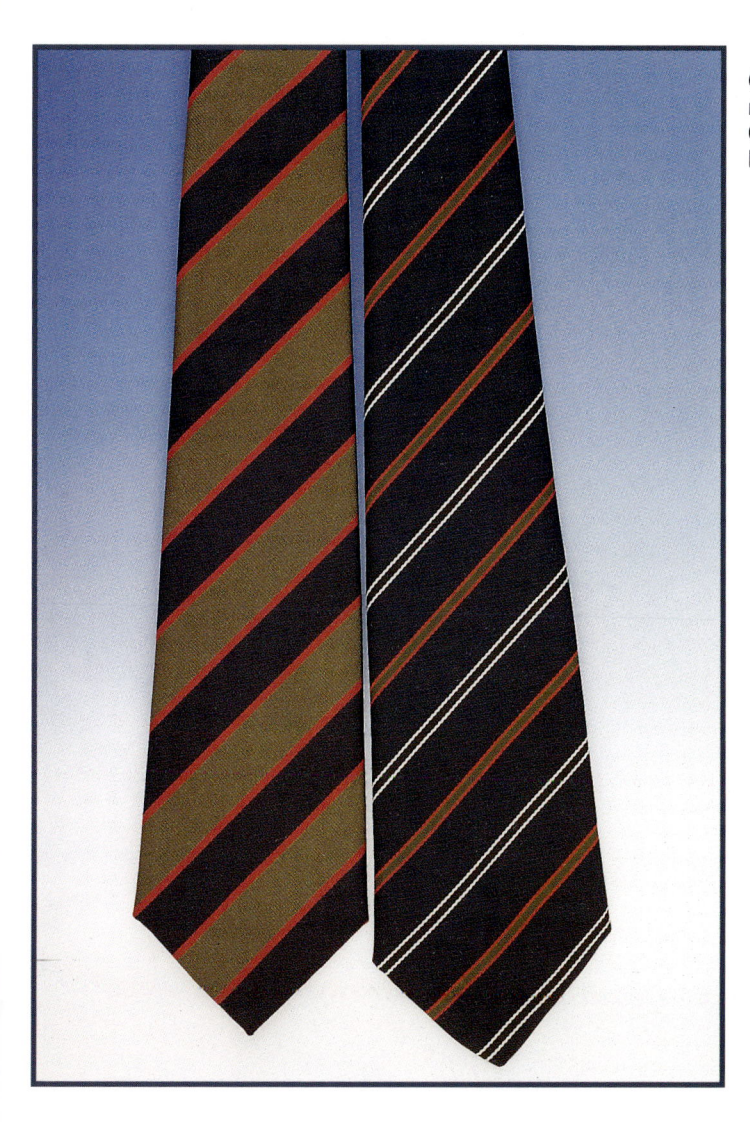

Queen's Royal Regiment (West Surrey); Queen's Royal Surrey Regiment (East & West)

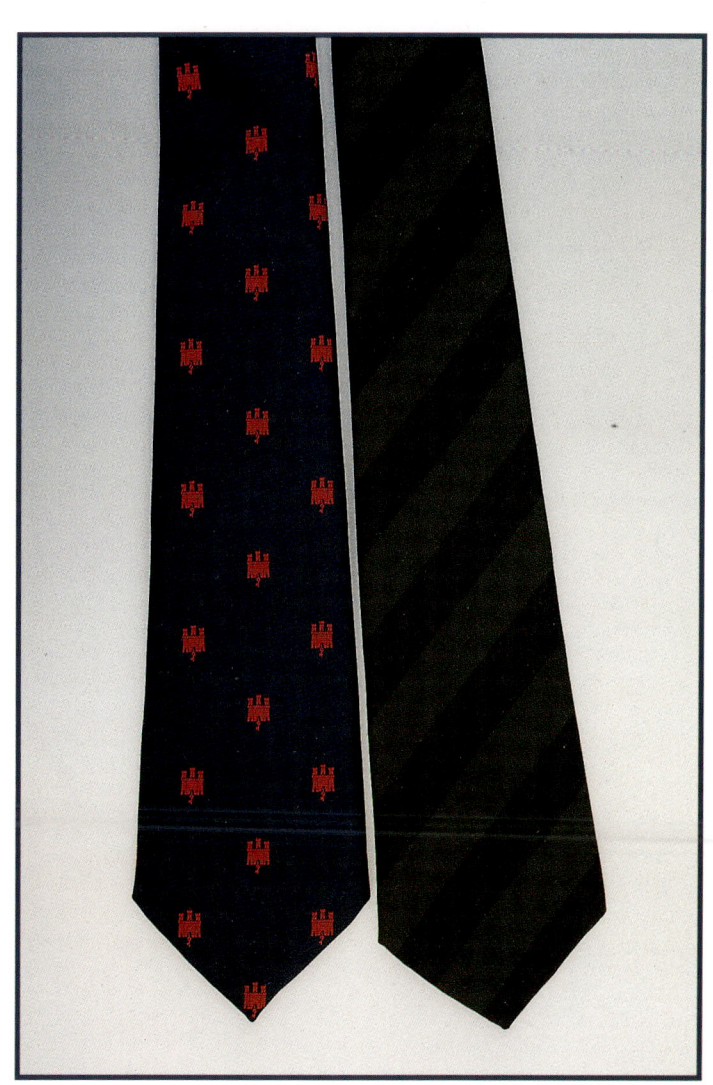

Royal Anglian Regiment; Rifle Brigade (Prince Consort's Own)

33

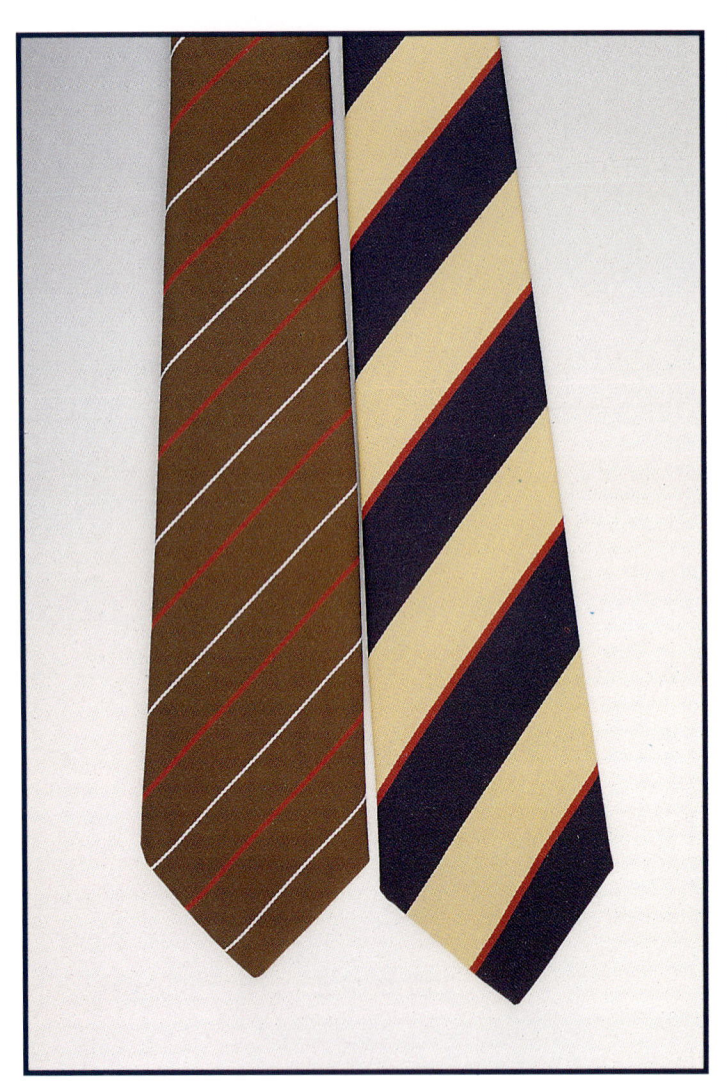

Royal Berkshire Regiment (Prince Charlotte of Wales's); Royal Gloucestershire, Berkshire and Wiltshire Regiment

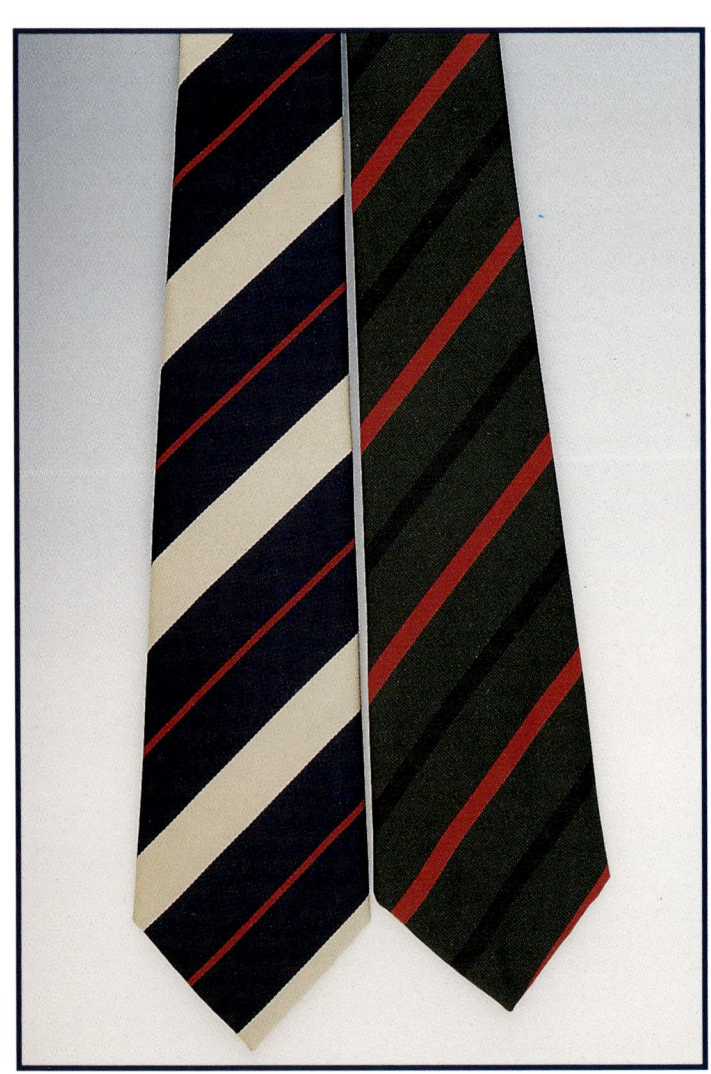

Royal Gloucestershire Hussars; Royal Green Jackets

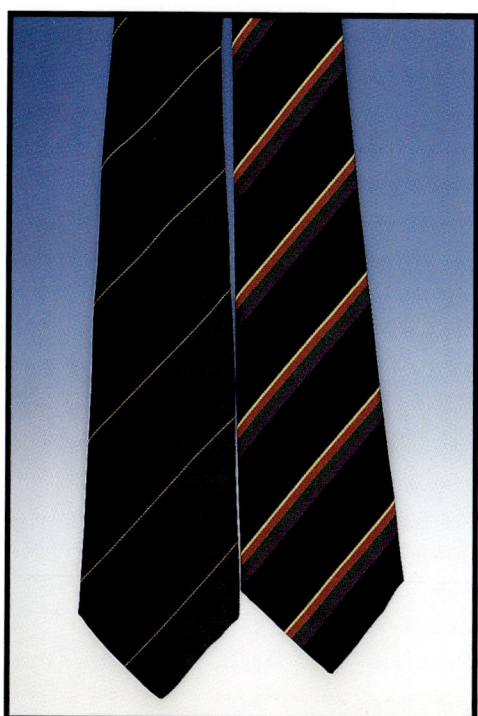

Royal Highland Fusiliers;
Royal Hampshire Regiment

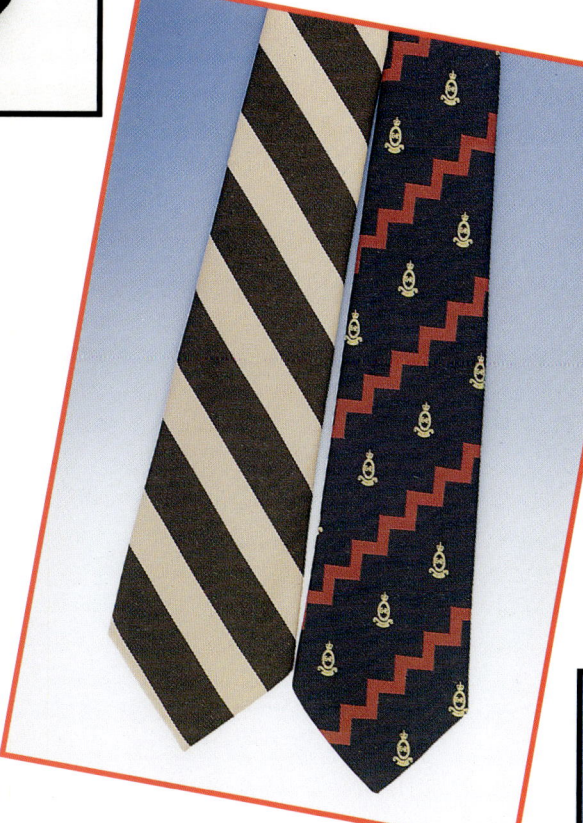

Royal Inniskilling
Fusiliers; Royal Horse
Artillery

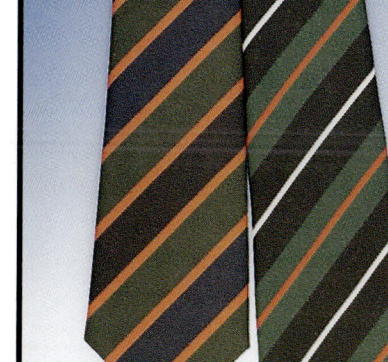

Royal Irish Fusiliers
(Princess Victoria's); Royal
Irish Rangers

35

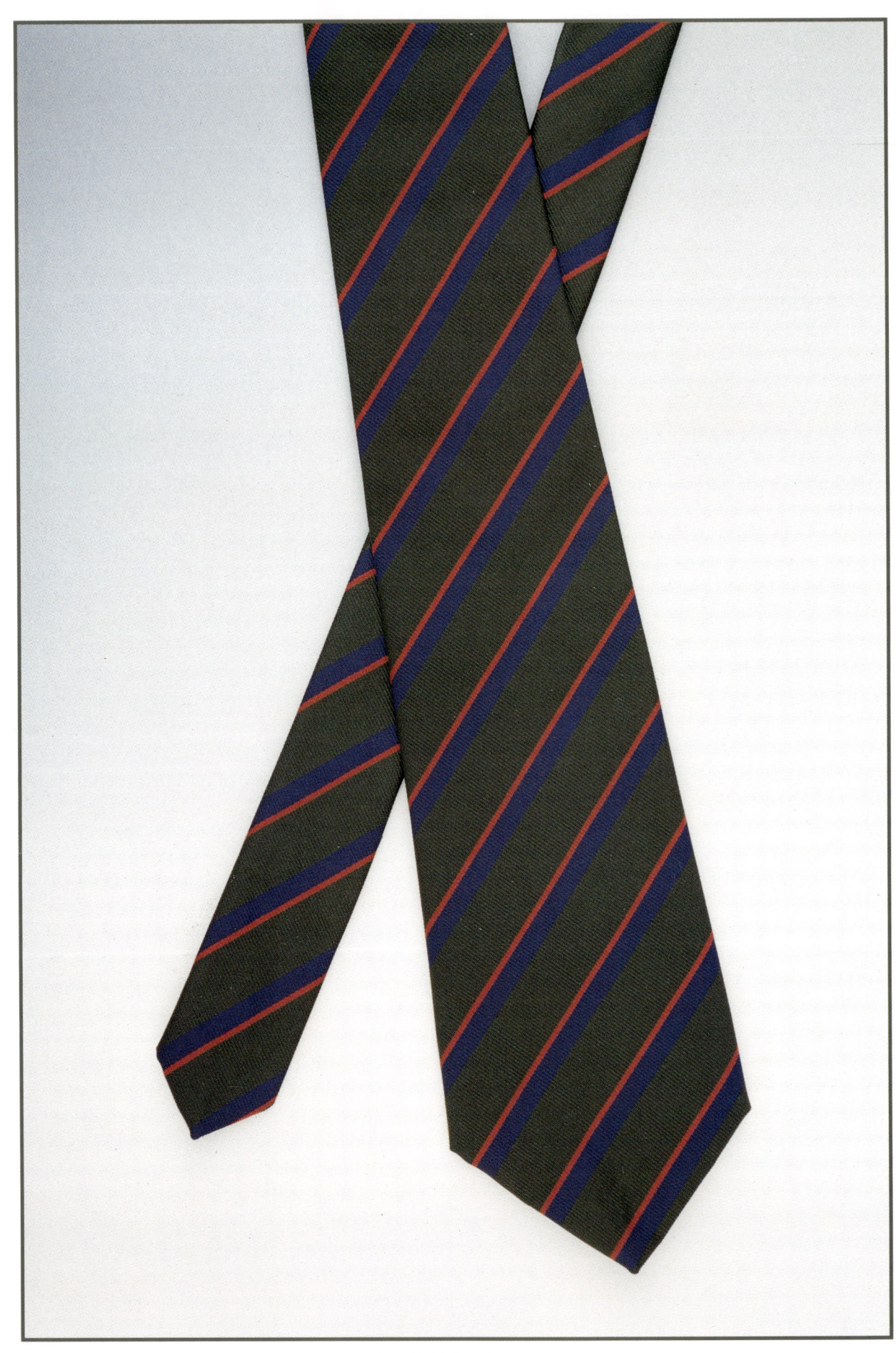

Royal Irish Regiment

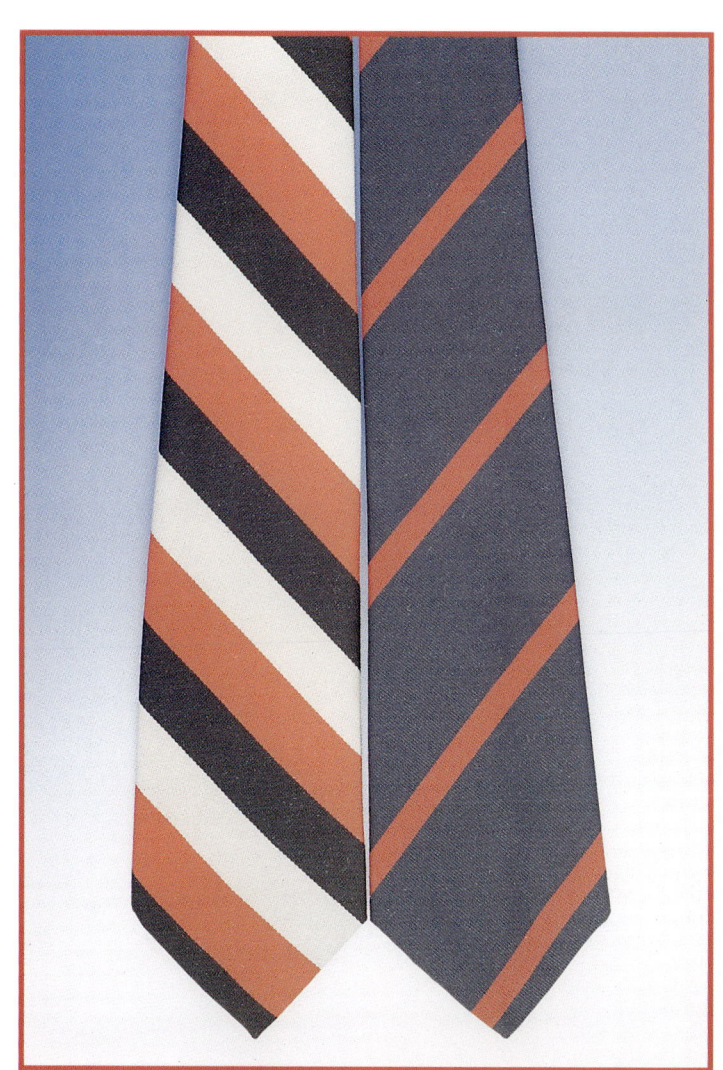

Royal Lincolnshire
Regiment; Royal
Leicestershire Regiment

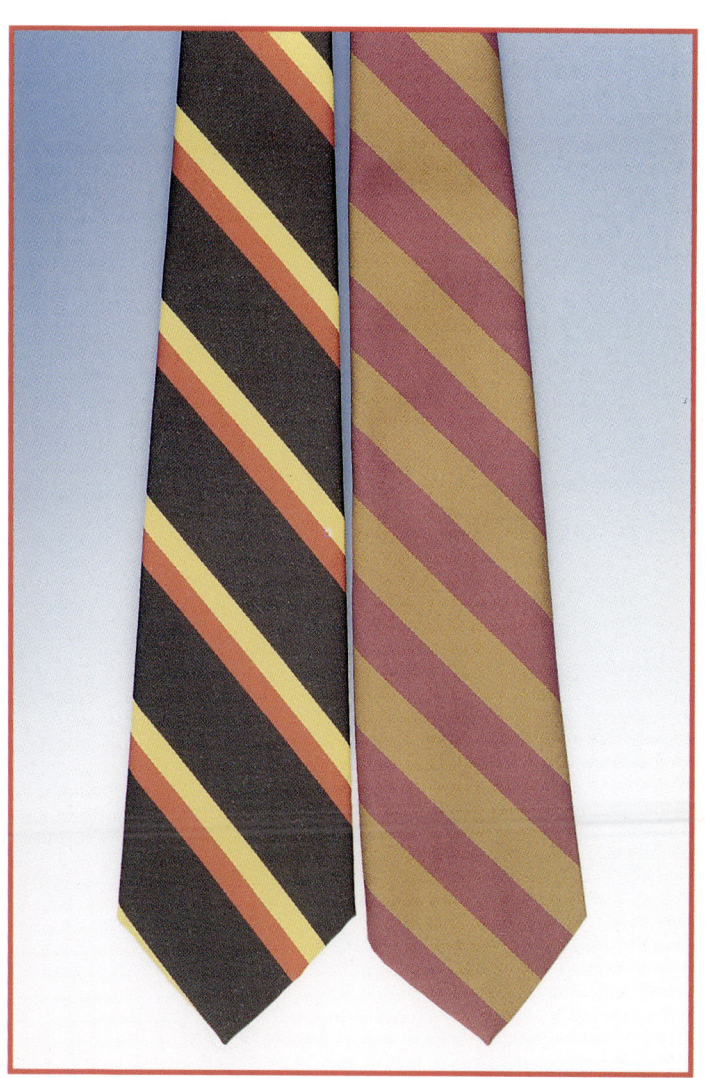

Royal Norfolk
Regiment; Royal
Northumberland
Fusiliers

37

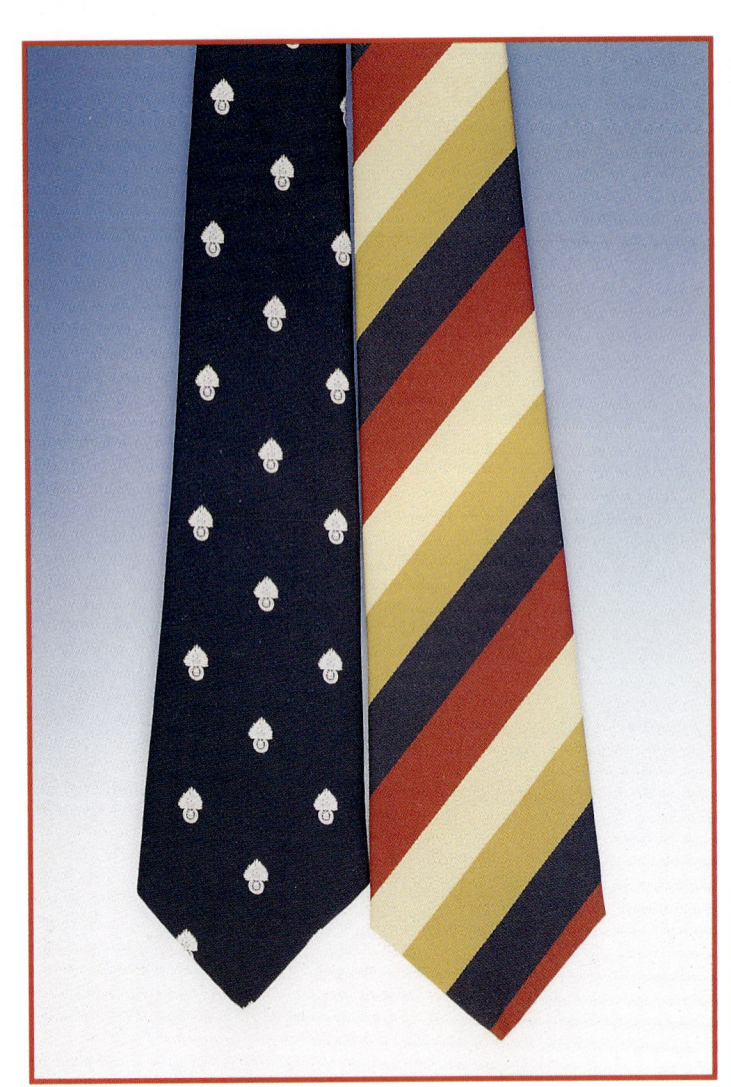

Royal Regiment of Fusiliers, crest and stripe

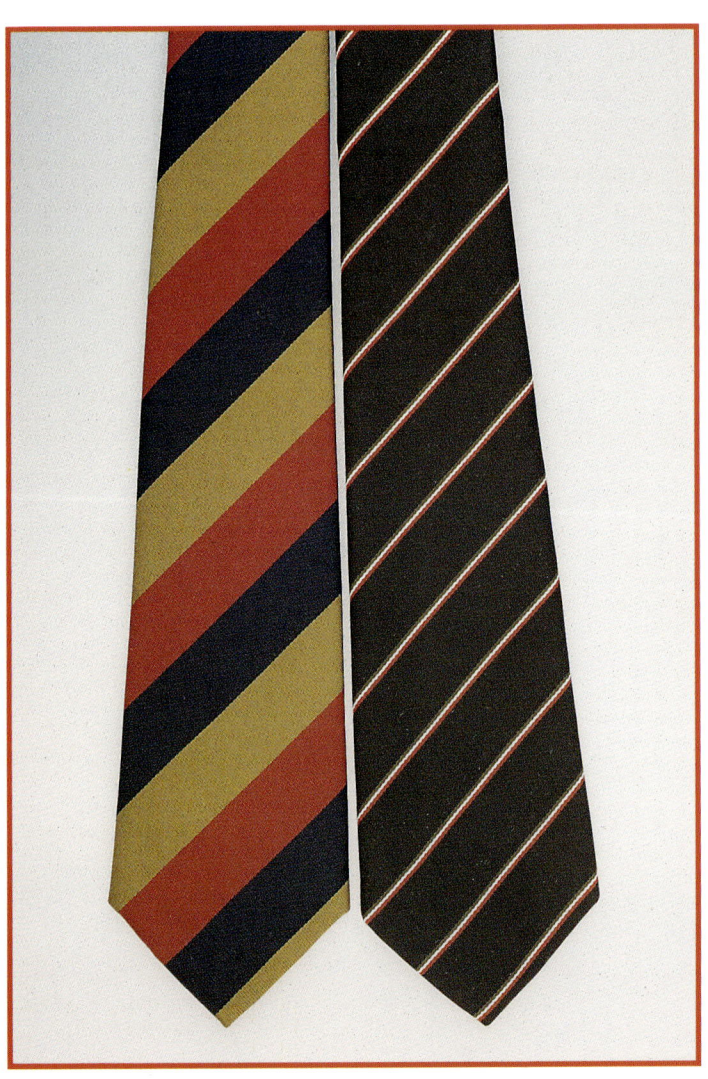

Royal Scots (Royal Regiment); Royal Regiment of Wales

38

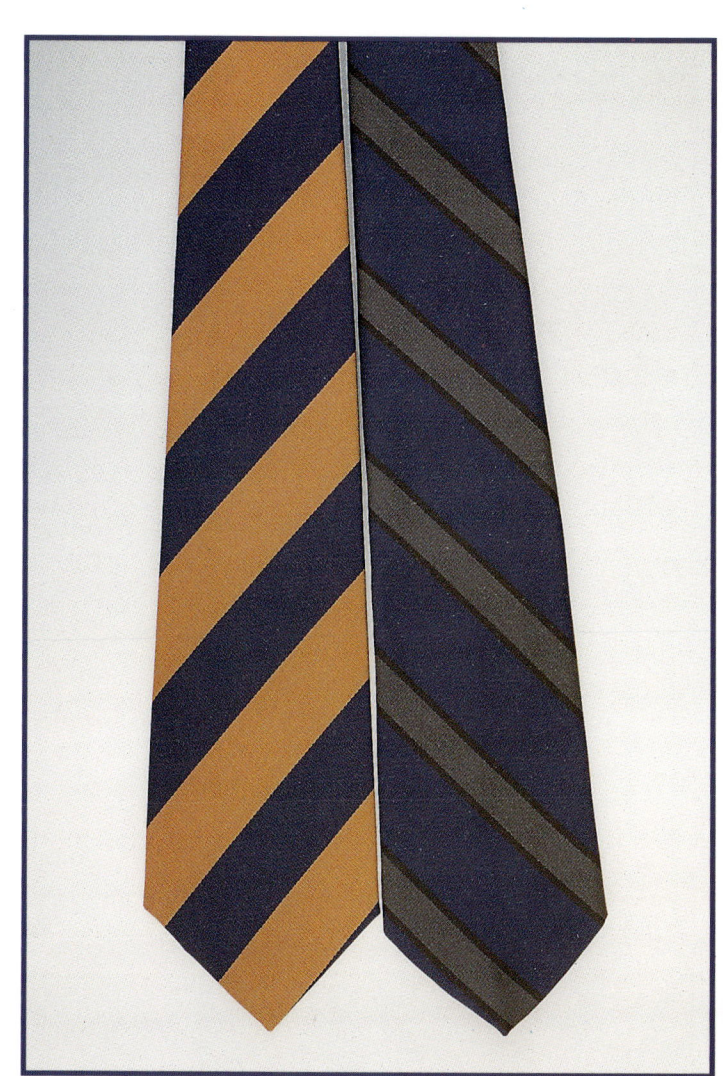

Royal Sussex Regiment;
Royal Scots Fusiliers

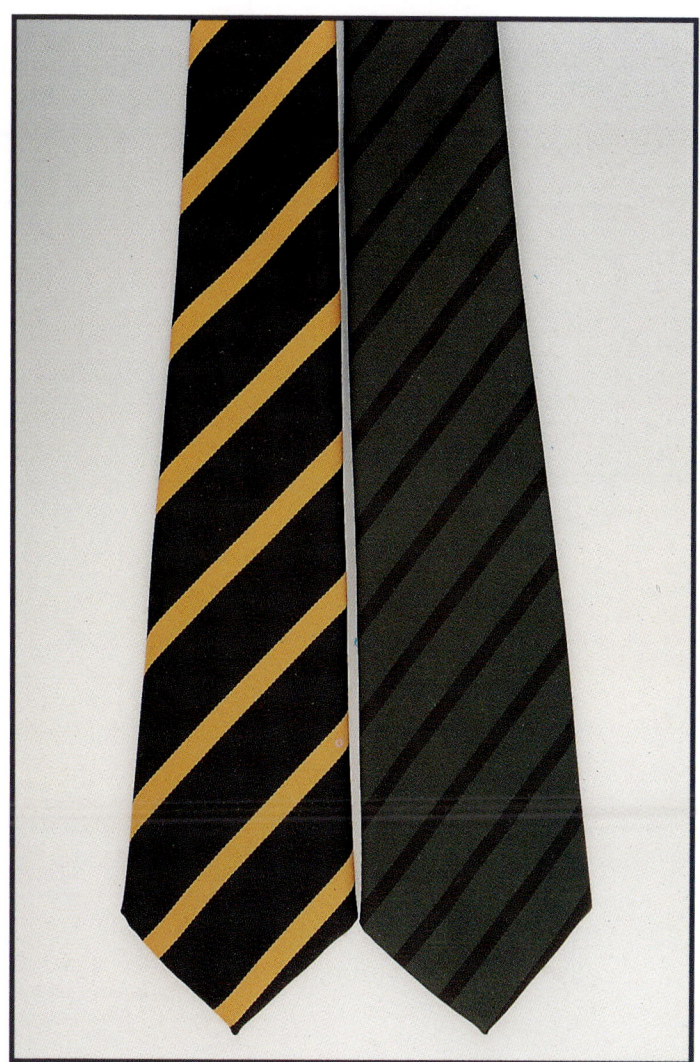

Royal Warwickshire
Regiment (Royal
Warwickshre Fusiliers);
Royal Ulster Rifles

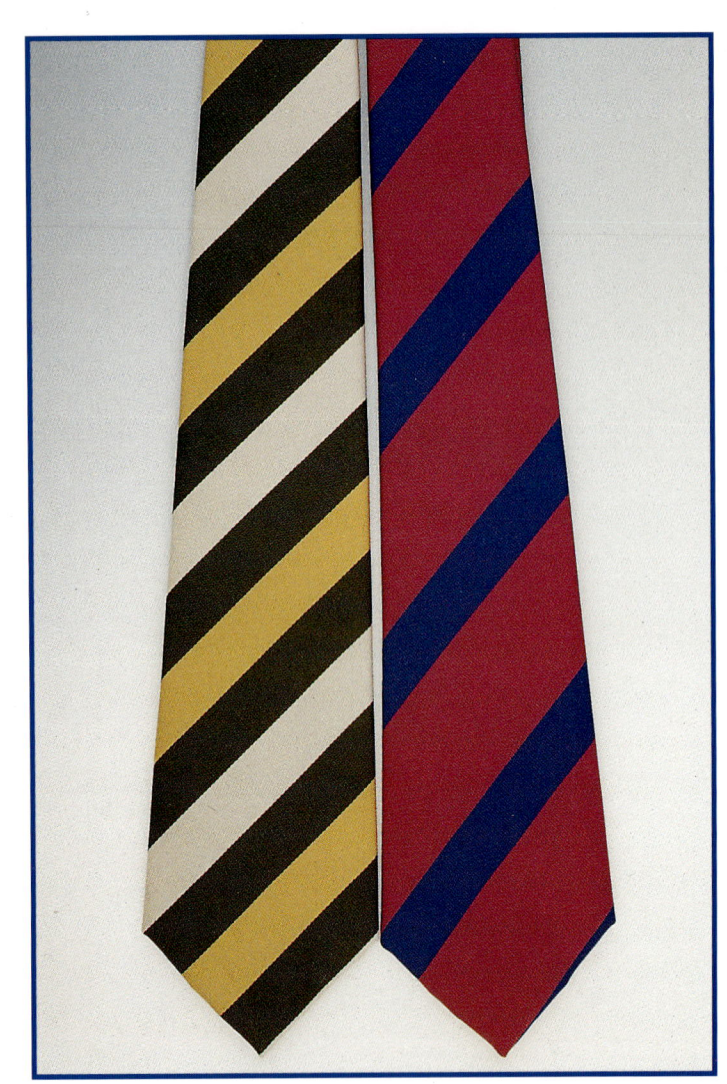

Royal Yeomanry; Royal Welch Fusiliers

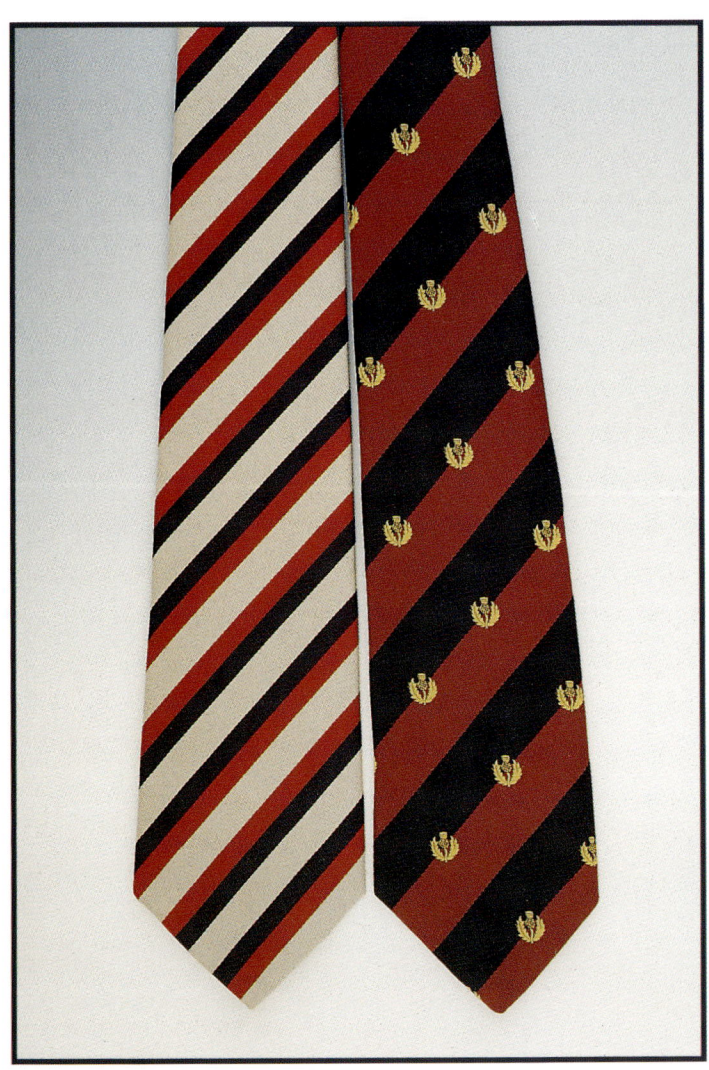

Seaforth Highlanders (Ross-shire Buffs, The Duke of Albany's); Scots Guards

40

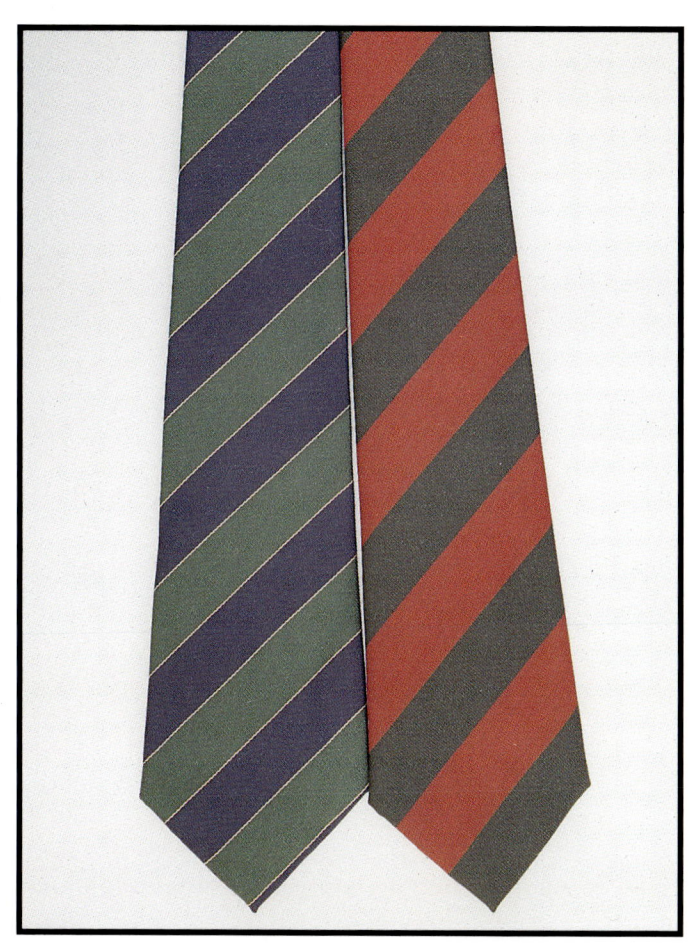

Somerset Light Infantry (Prince Albert's); Sherwood Foresters (Nottinghamshire and Derbyshire Regiment)

South Wales Borderers; South Staffordshire Regiment

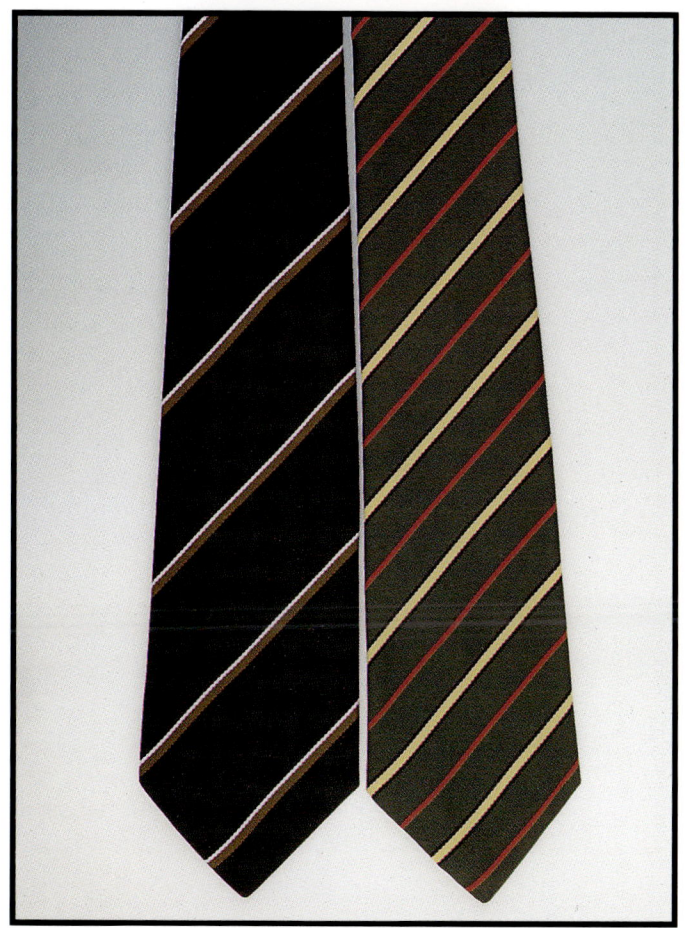

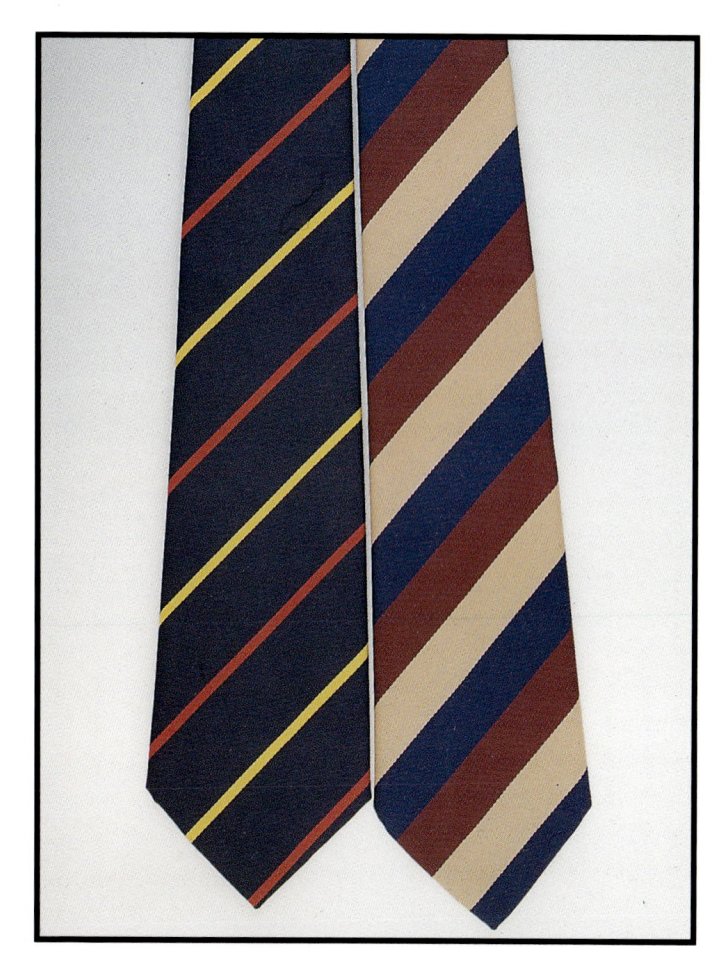

South Nottinghamshire Hussars; South Lancashire Regiment (The Prince of Wales's Volunteers)

Suffolk Regiment; Staffordshire Regiment (The Prince of Wales's)

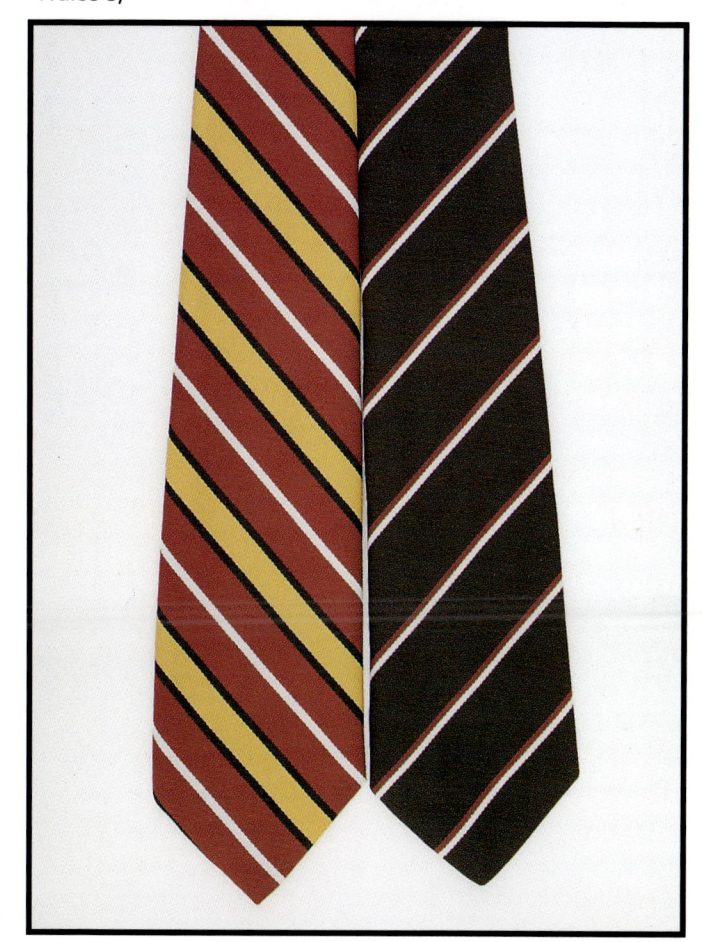

41

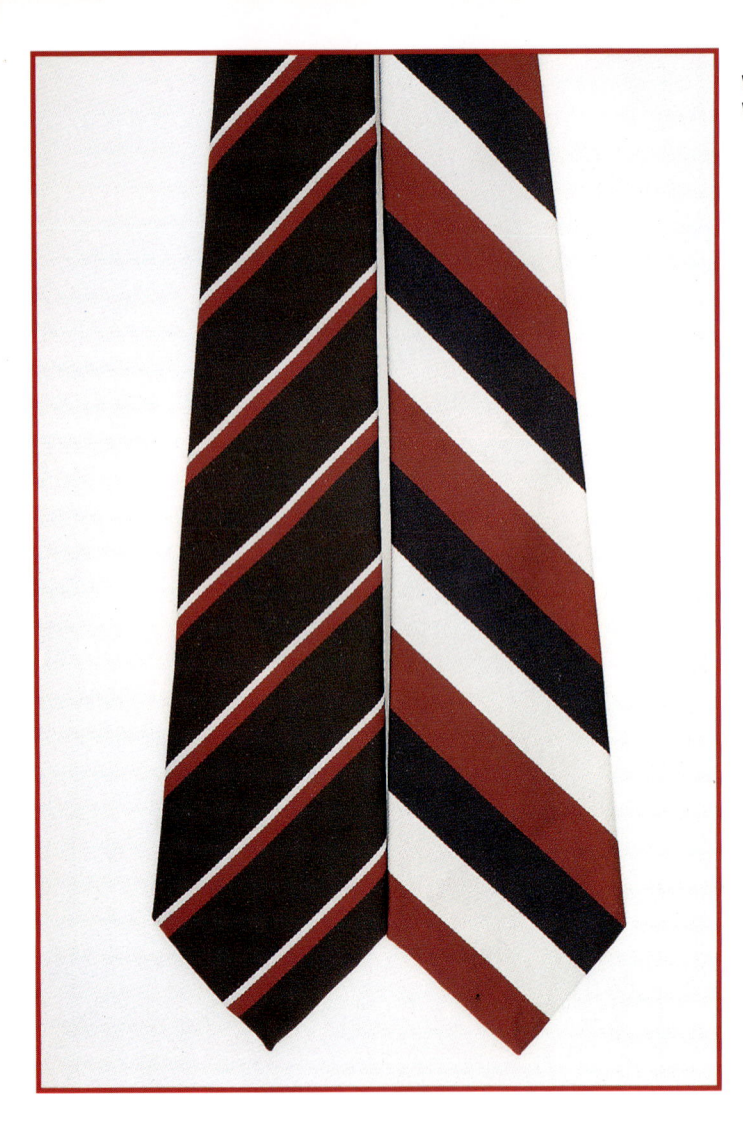

Welsh Regiment;
Warwickshire Yeomanry

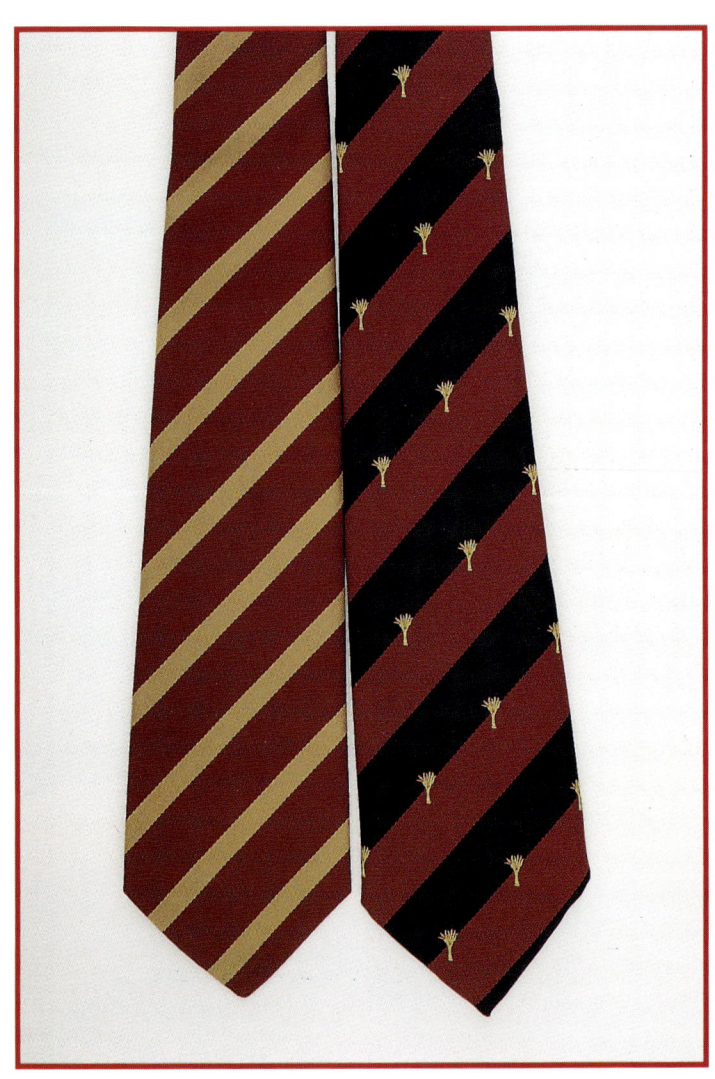

West Yorkshire Regiment
(The Prince of Wales's
Own); Welsh Guards

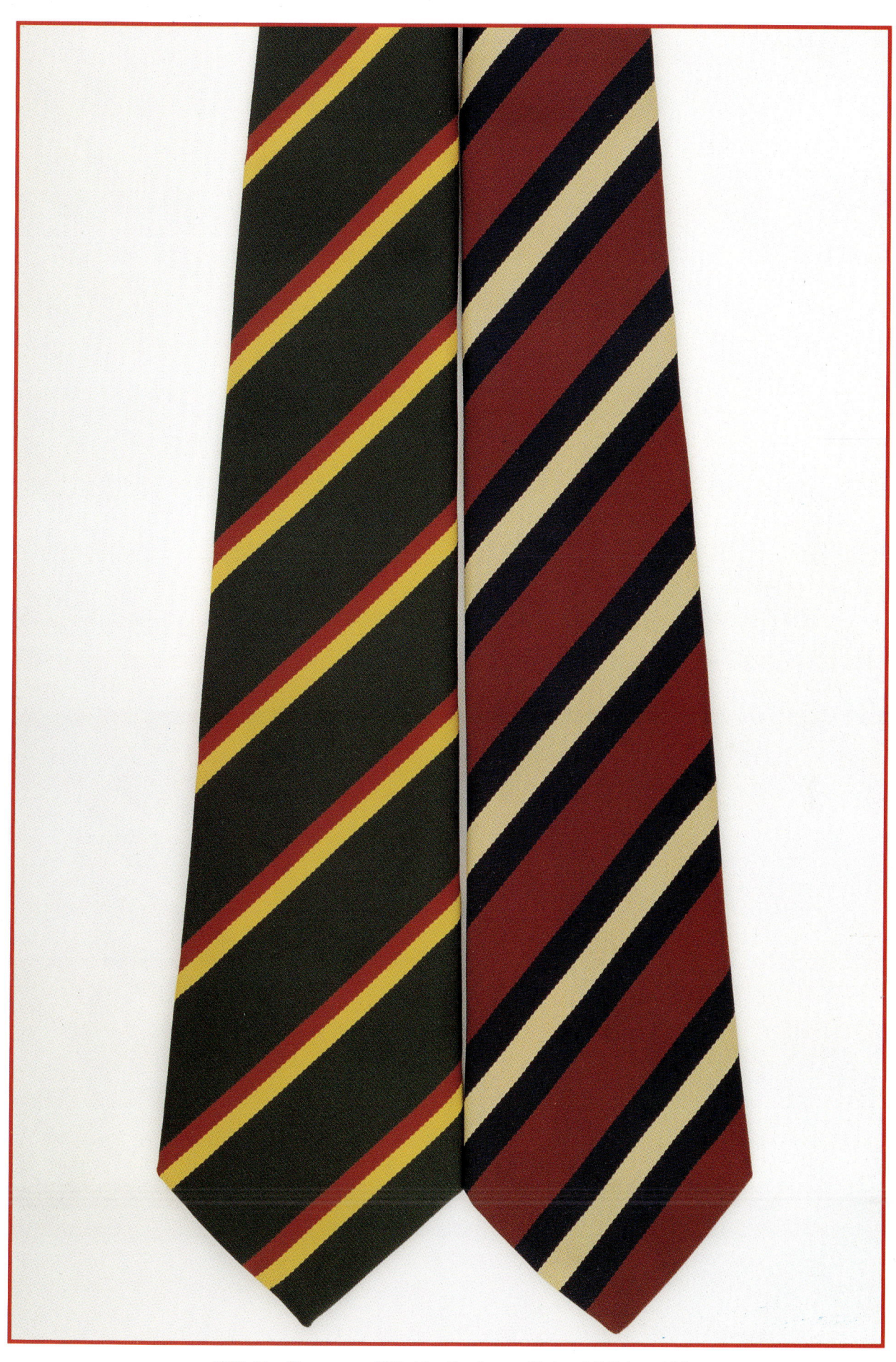

Wiltshire Yeomanry; Wiltshire Regiment (Duke of Edinburgh's)

43

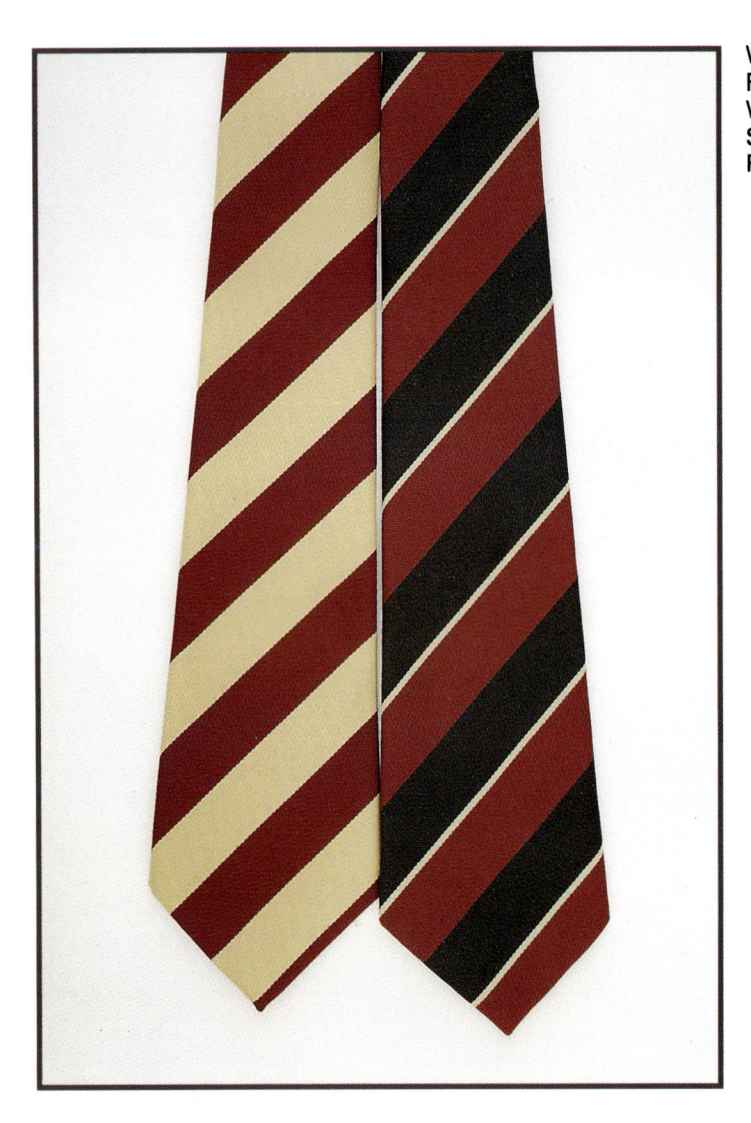

Worcestershire
Regiment;
Worcestershire and
Sherwood Foresters
Regiment

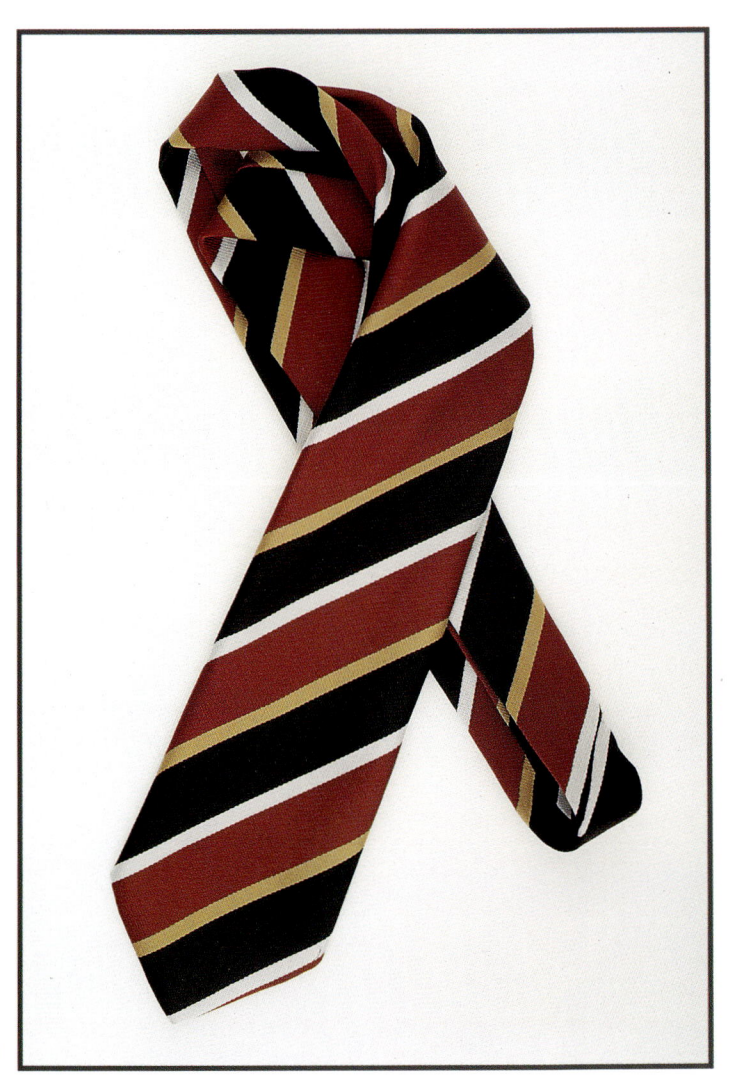

York and Lancaster
Regiment

44

Gurkha, Indian, and Colonial

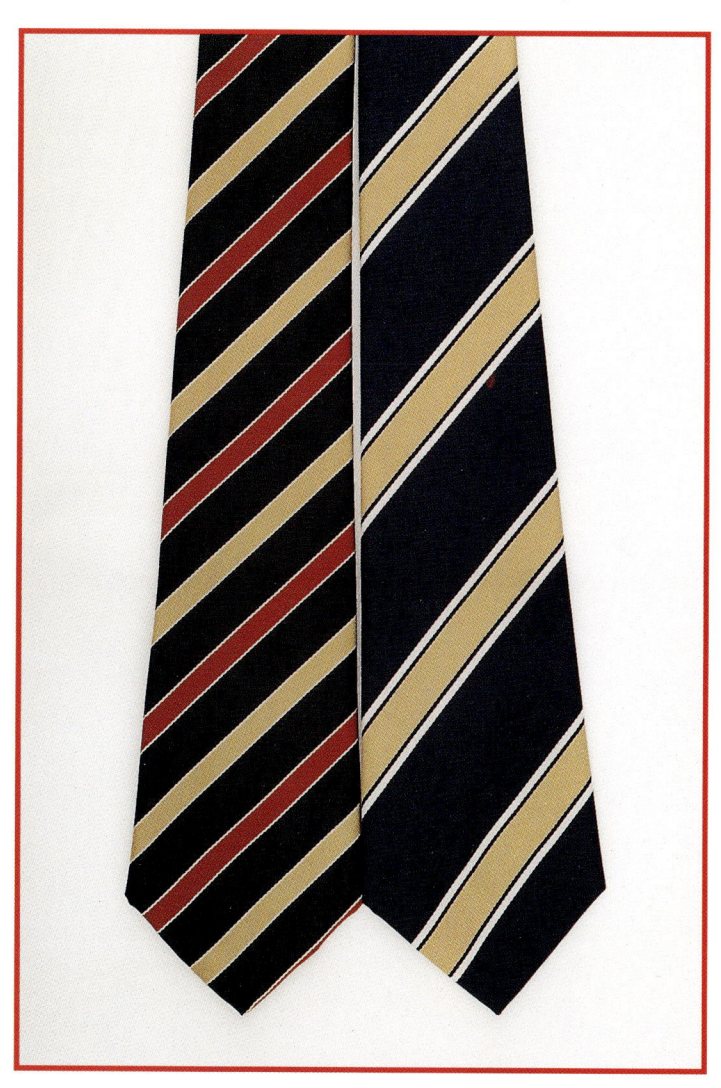

Calcutta Light Horse; Assam Valley Light Horse

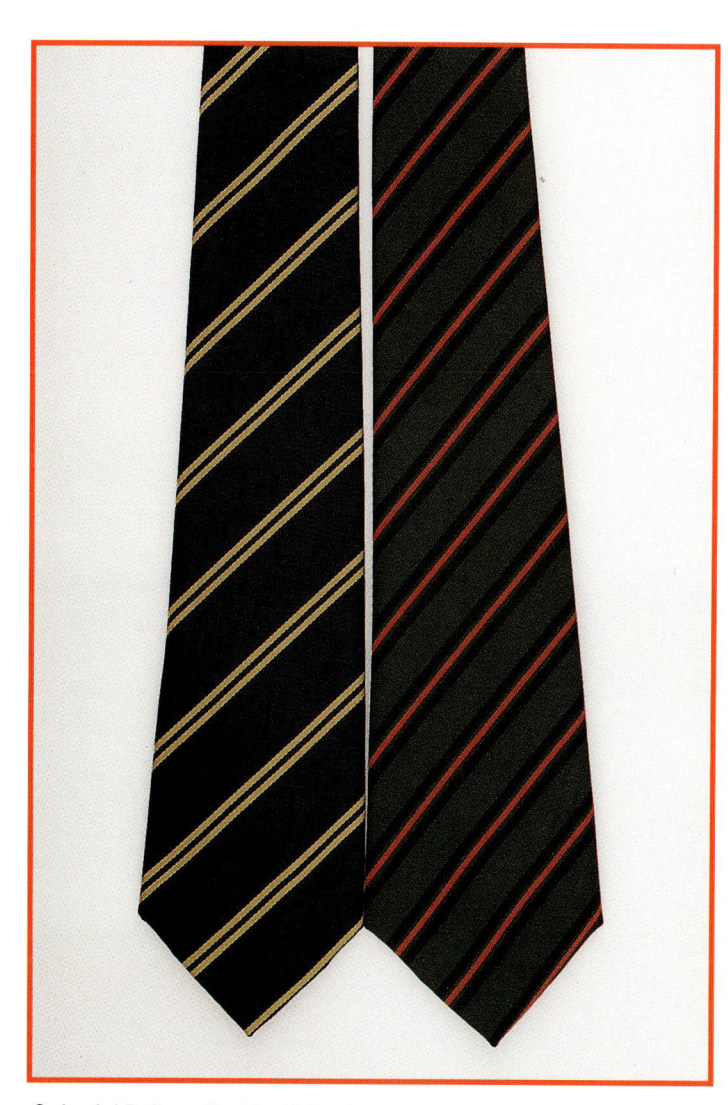

Colonial Police; Gurkha Brigade

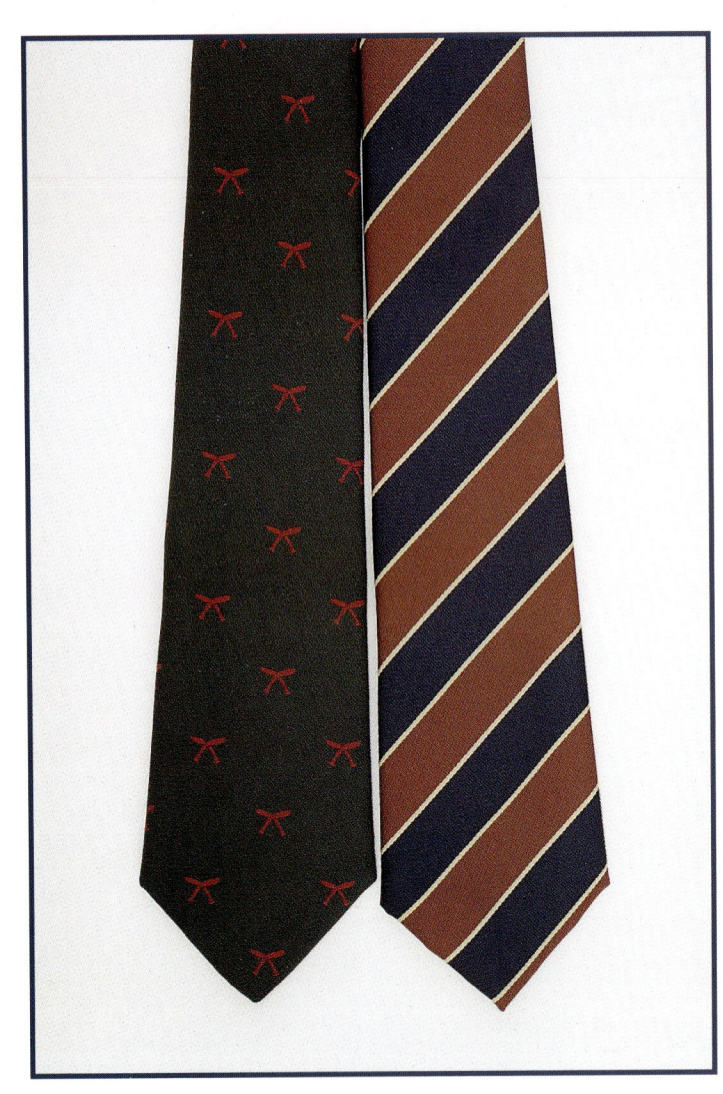

Gurkha Brigade; Indian Army General

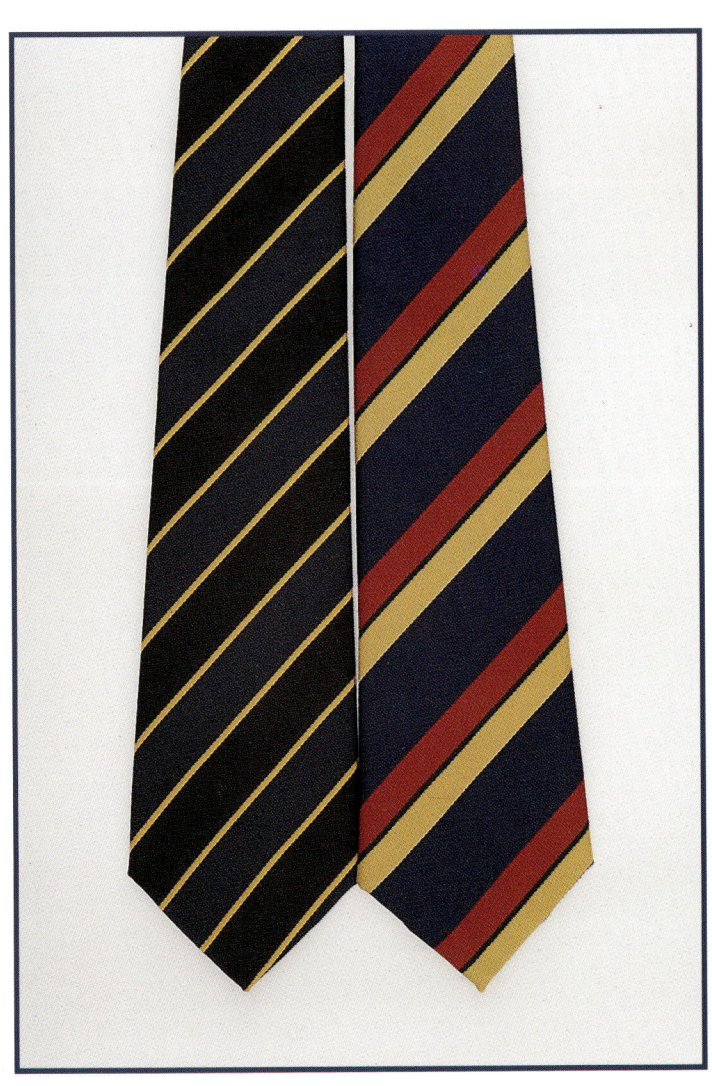

King's African Rifles; Kenya Police

46

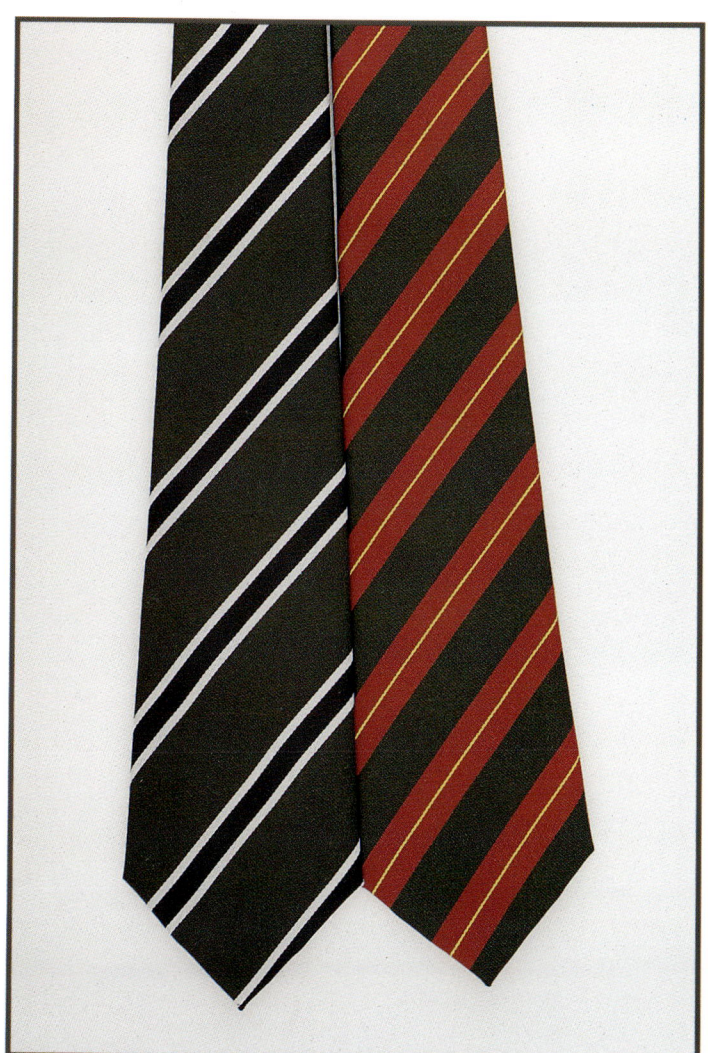

Nigeria Regiment; Punjab Frontier Force

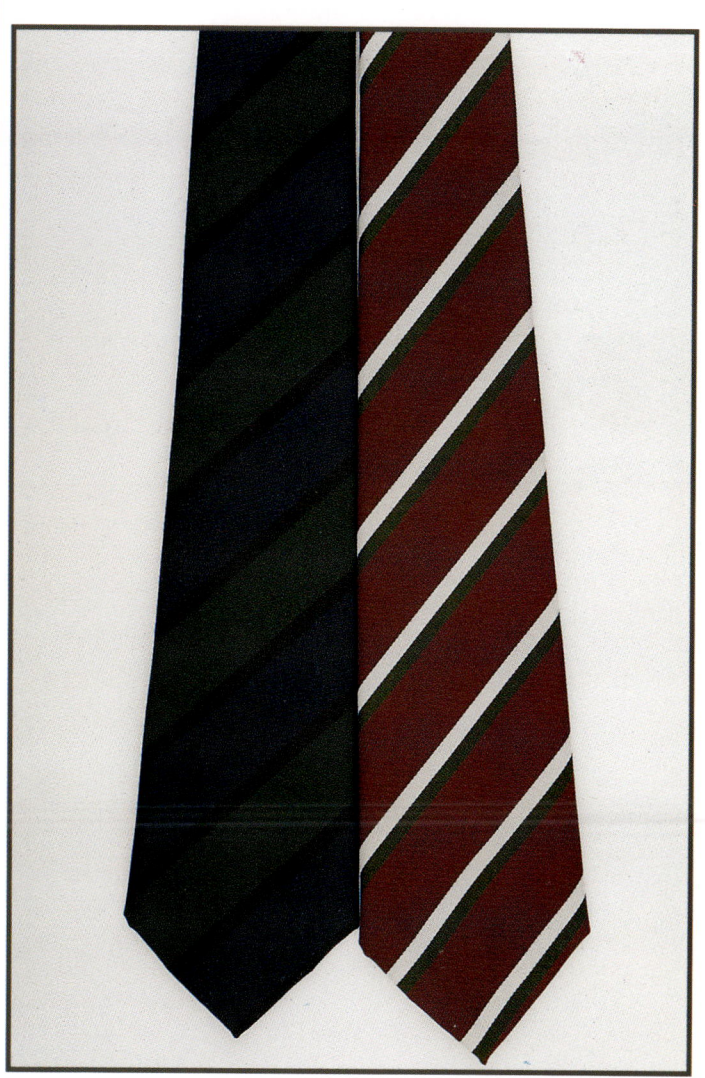

Royal West African Frontier Force; Staff College, Quetta

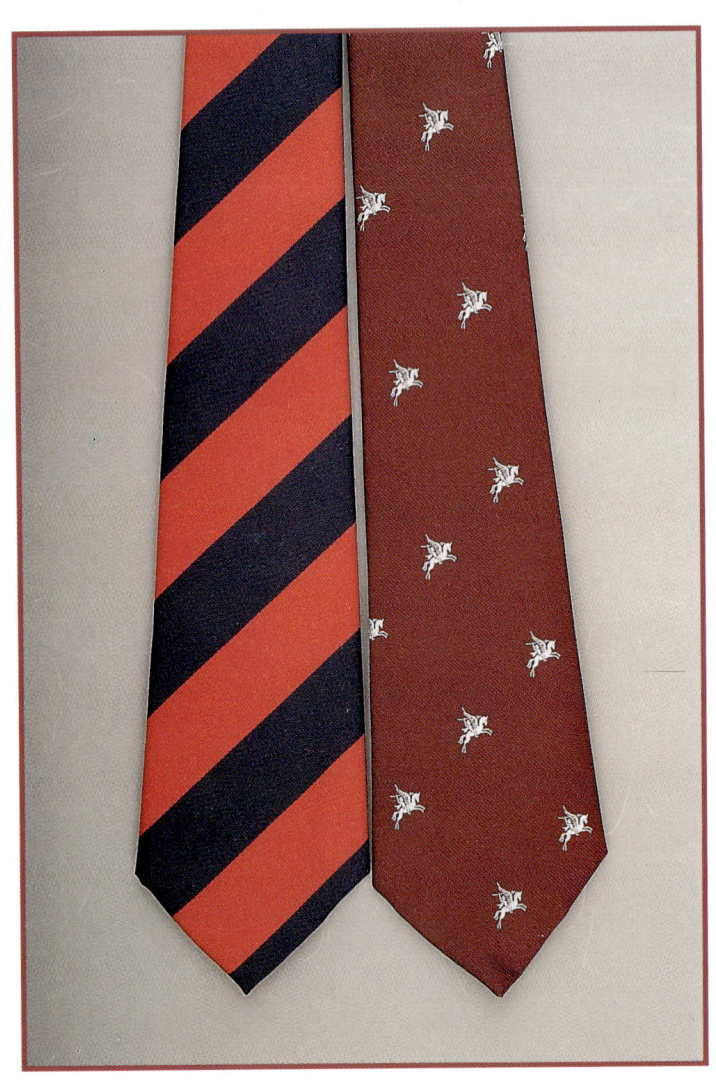

Adjutant General's Corps; Airborne Division

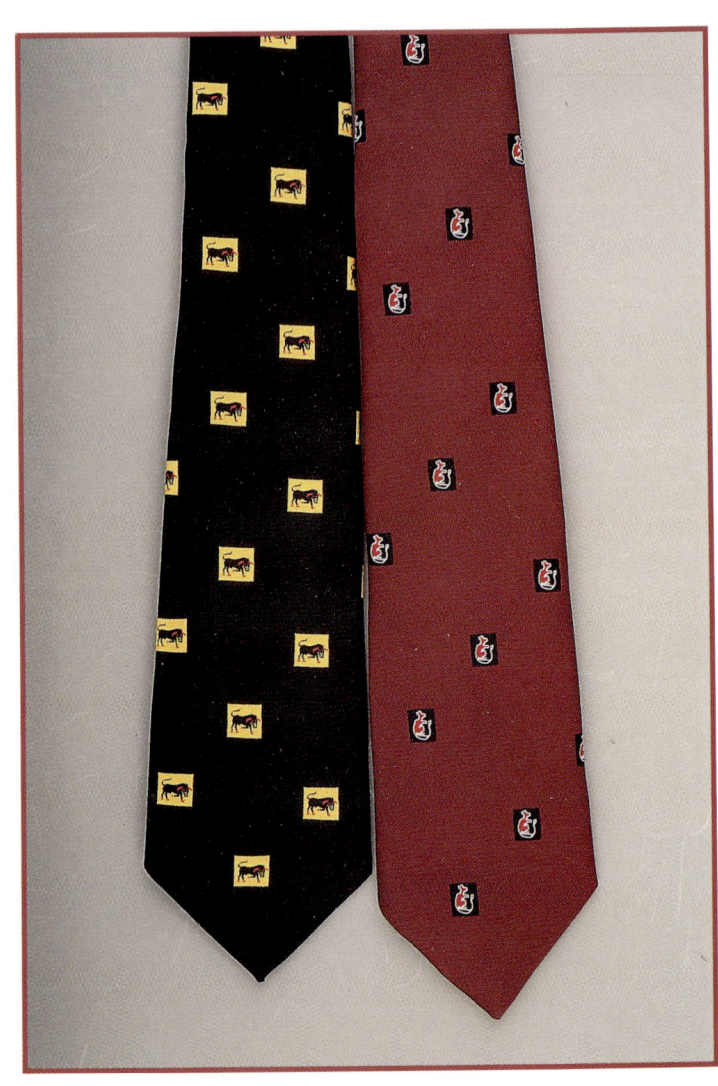

11th Armoured Division; 7th Armoured Division

48

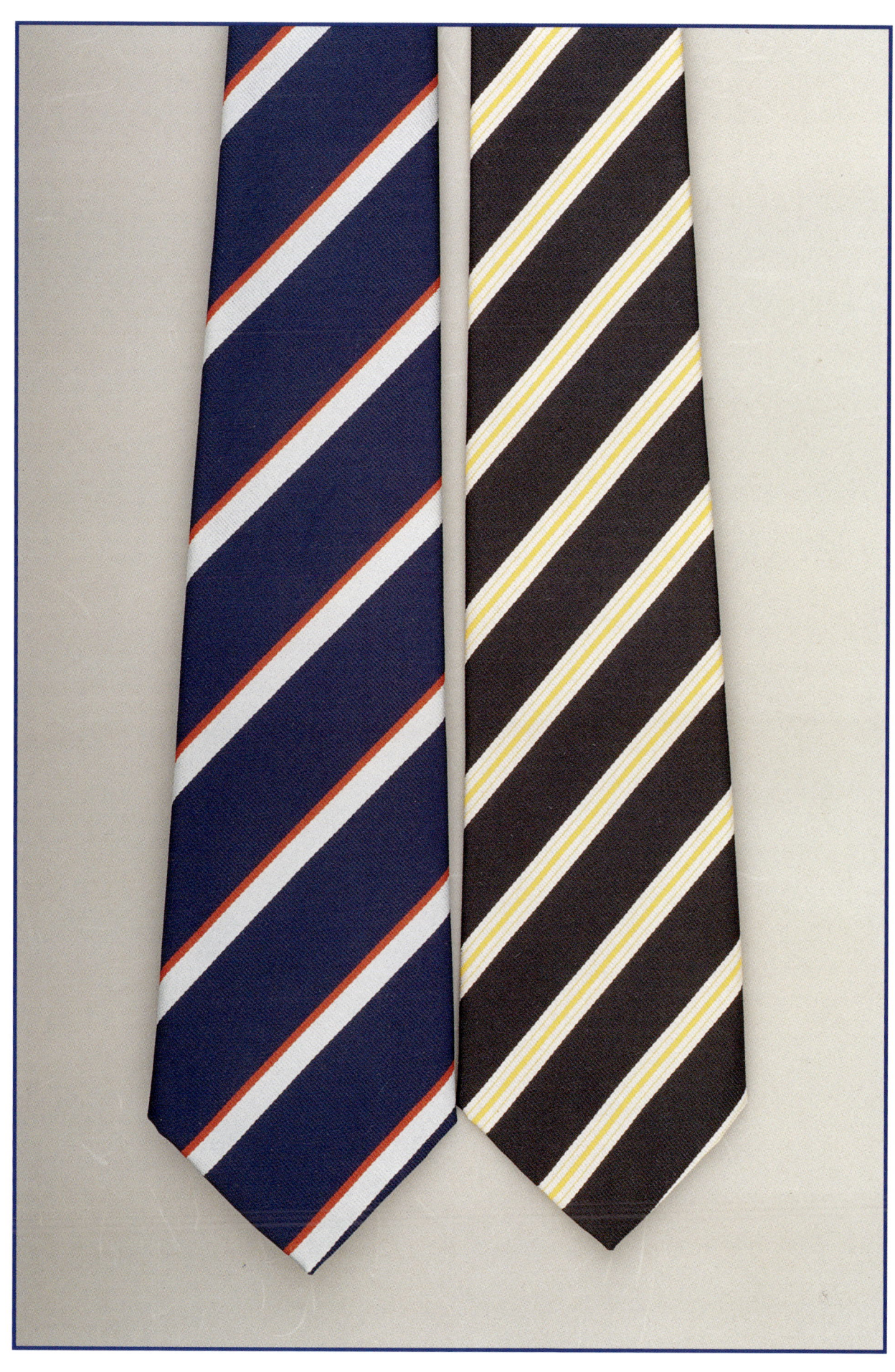

Army Air Corps; Army Catering Corps

Army Physical Training
Corps; 2nd Army

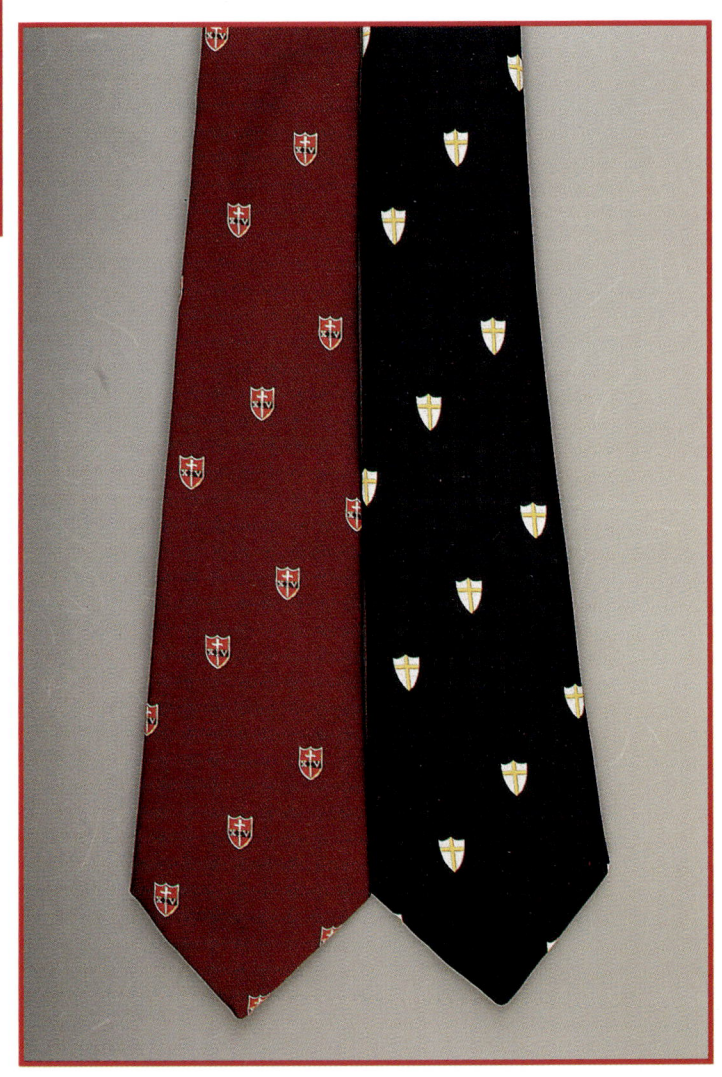

14th Army; 8th Army

50

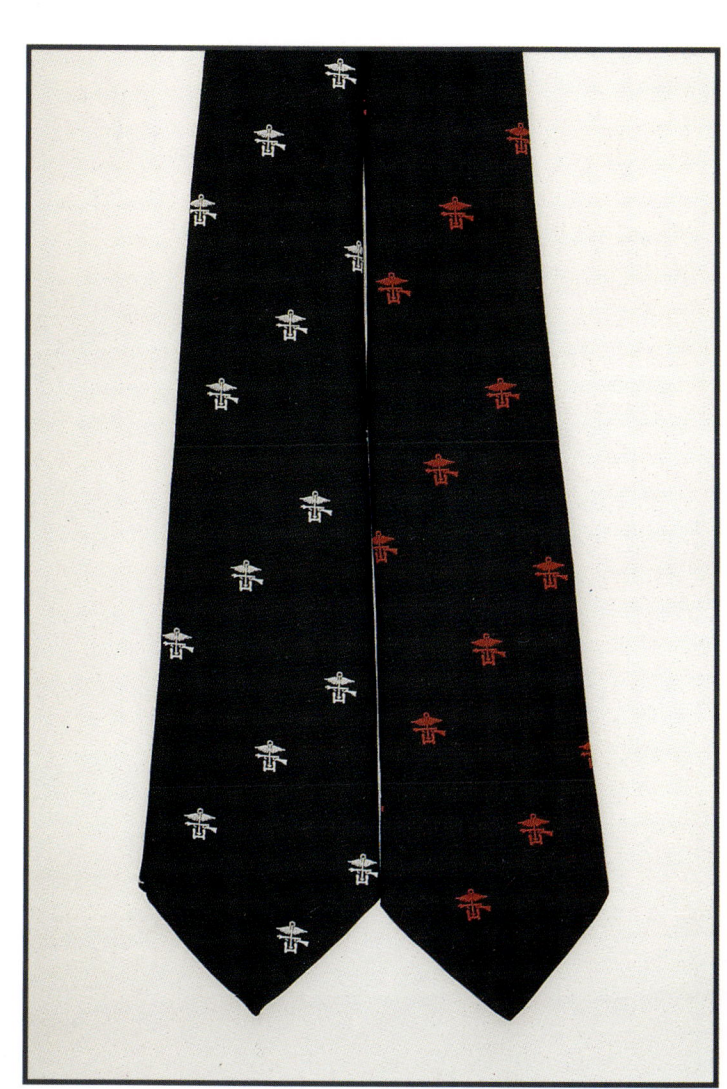

Combined Operations,
white and red motifs

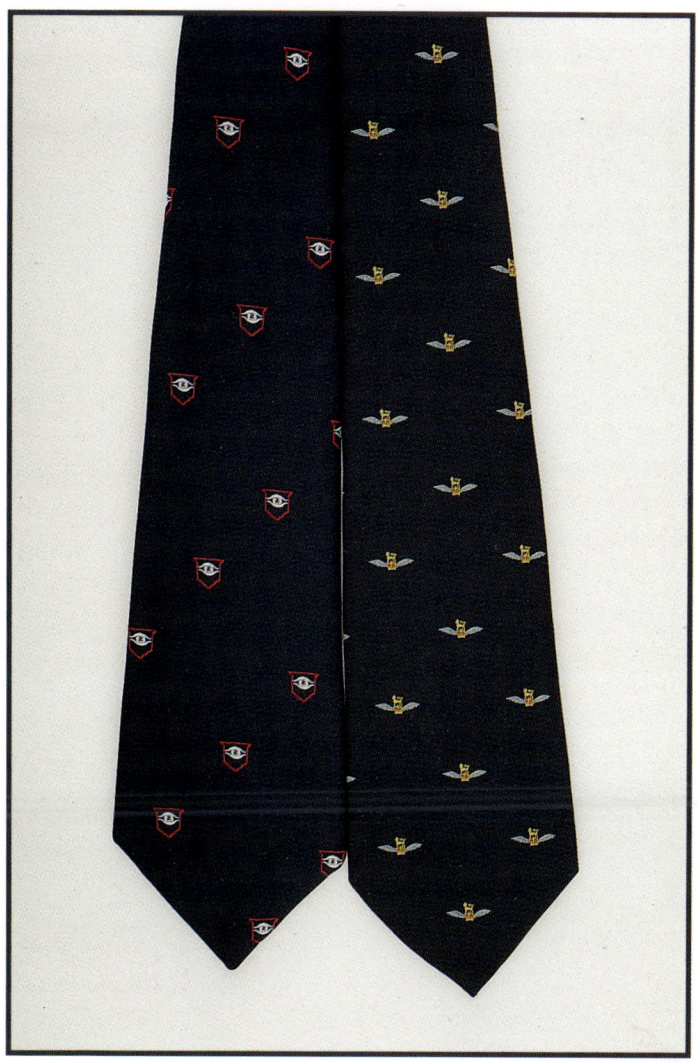

Guards Armoured Division;
Glider Pilots

51

2nd Infantry Division;
3rd Infantry Division

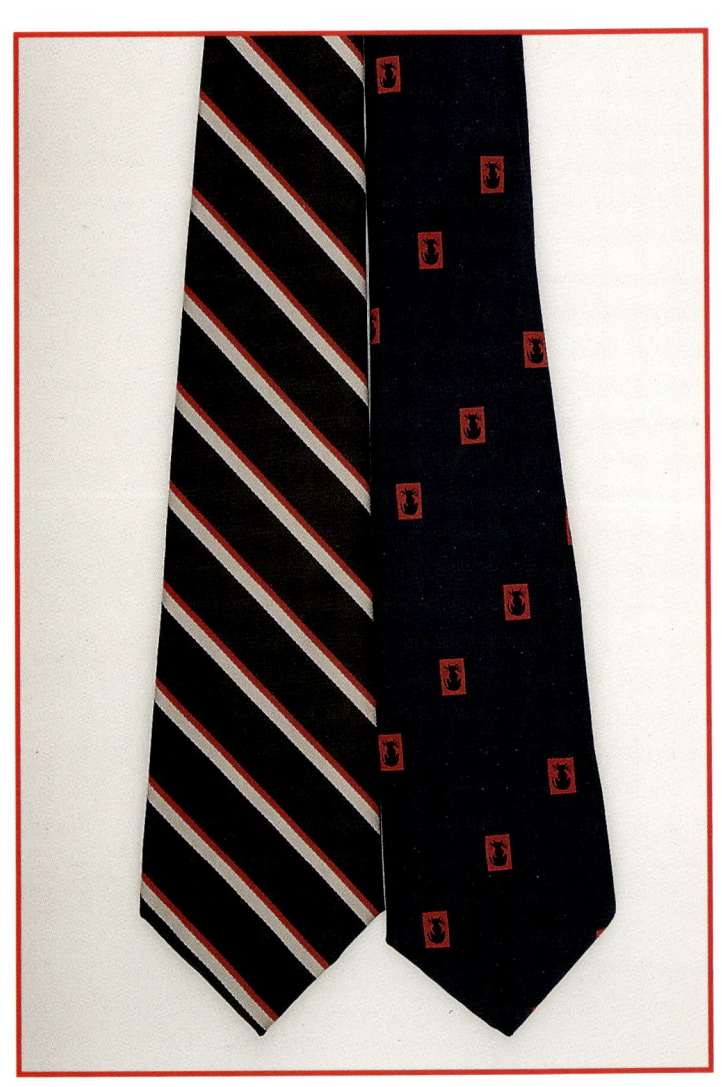

Intelligence Corps;
56th London Division

52

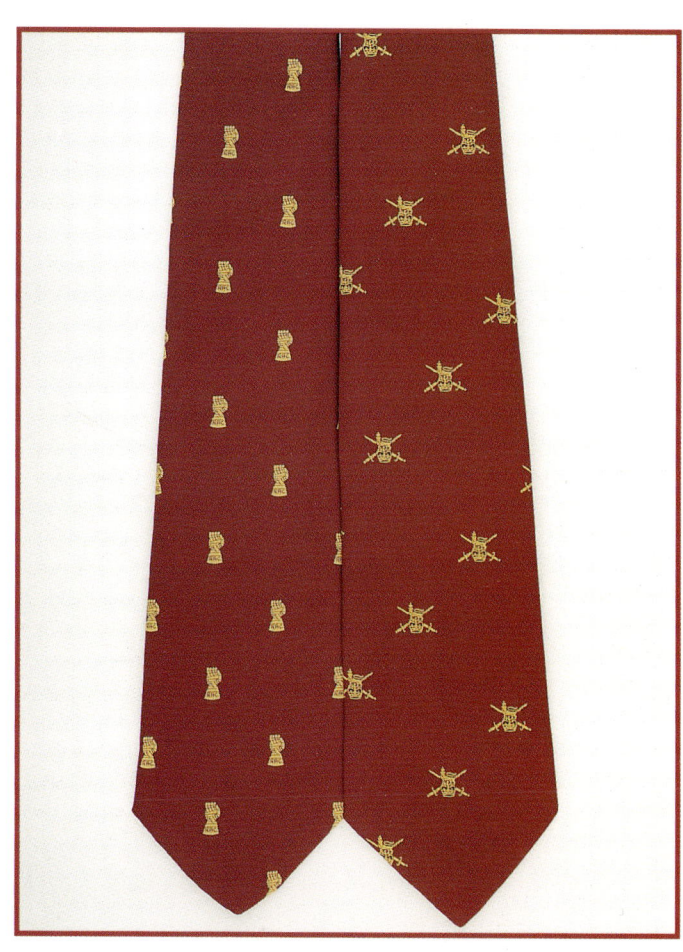

Royal Armoured Corps; Regular Army

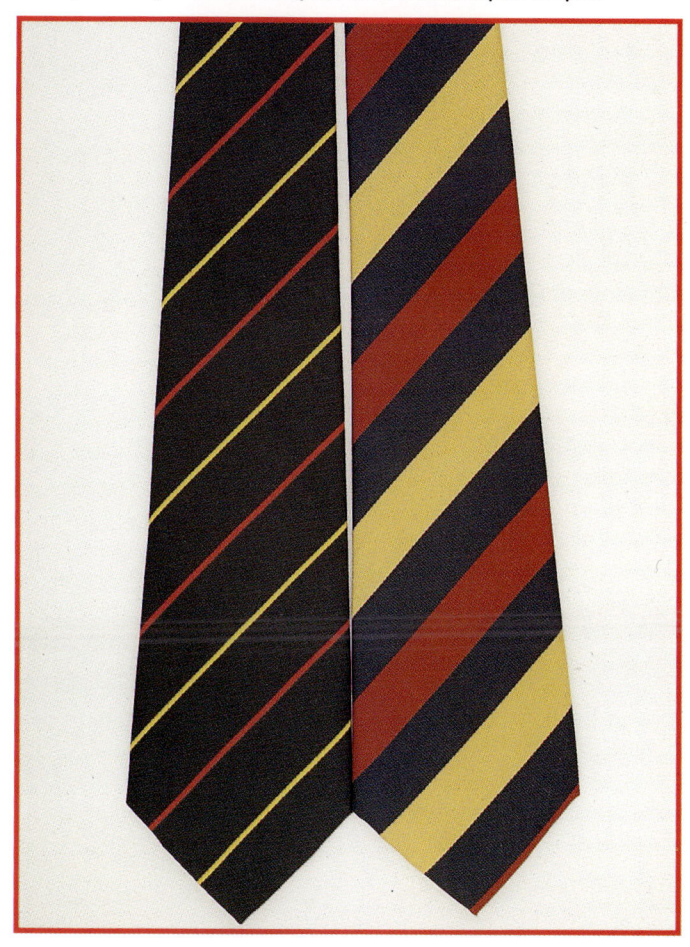

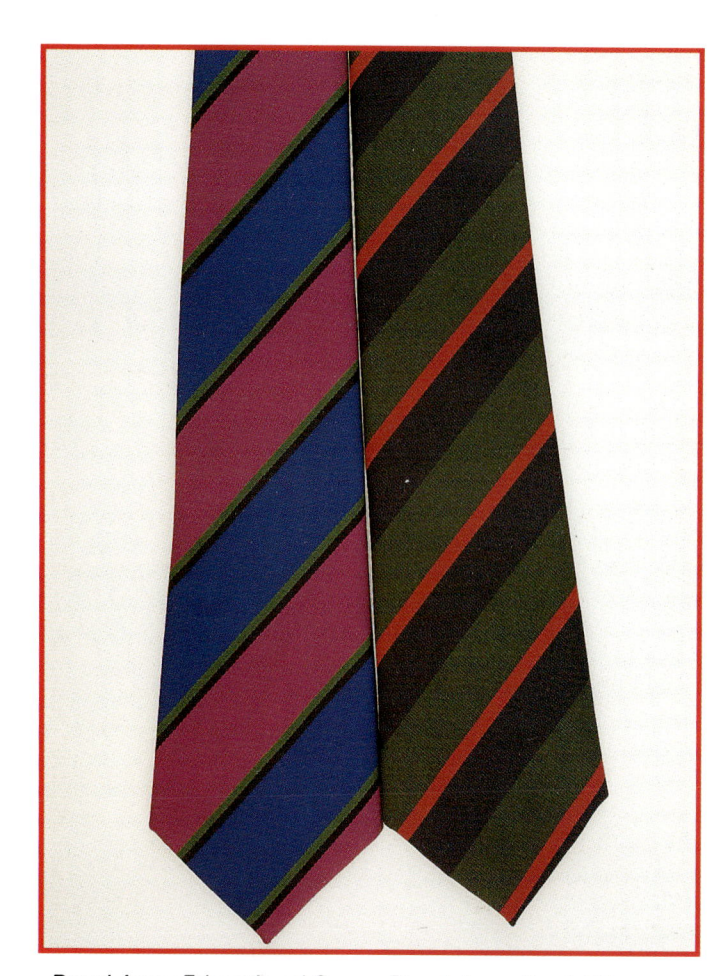

Royal Army Educational Corps; Royal Army Dental Corps

Royal Army Medical Corps, narrow and equal stripes

Royal Army Ordnance Corps (old pattern); Royal Army Medical Corps, crest

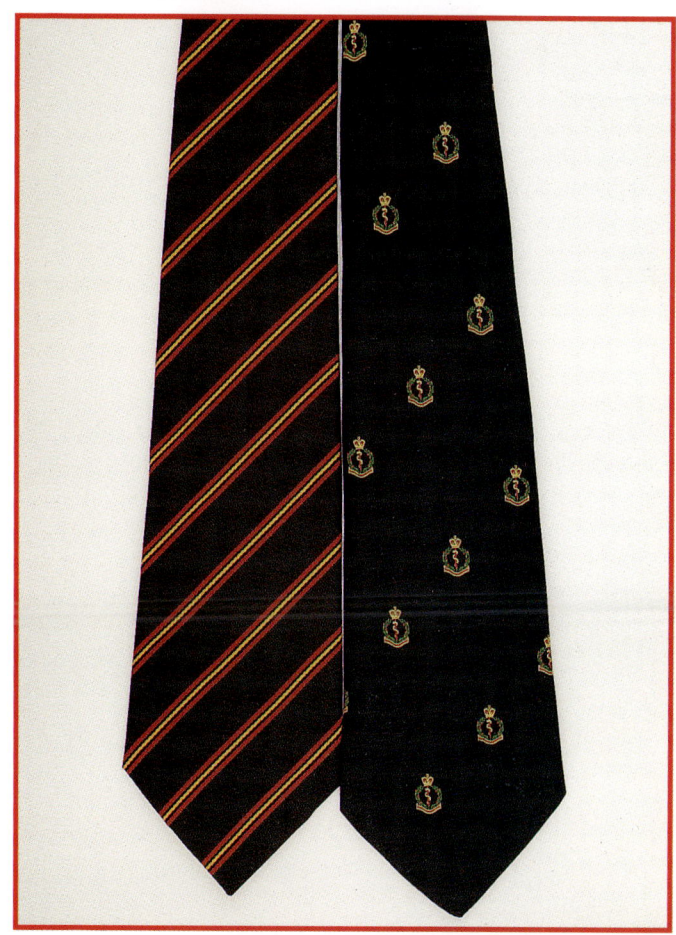

53

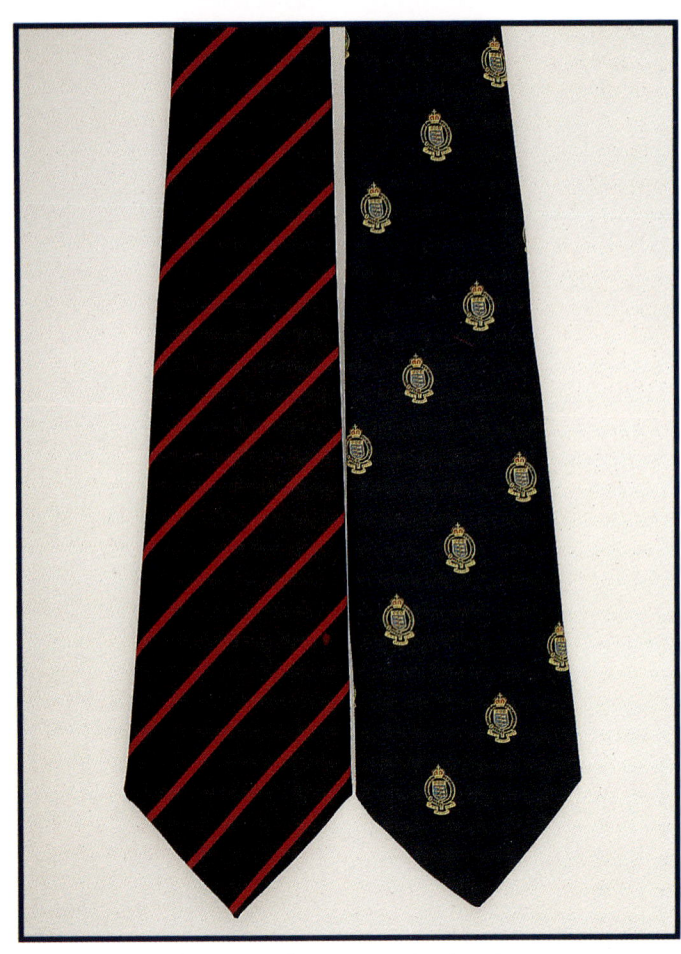

Royal Army Ordnance Corps, navy/red and crest

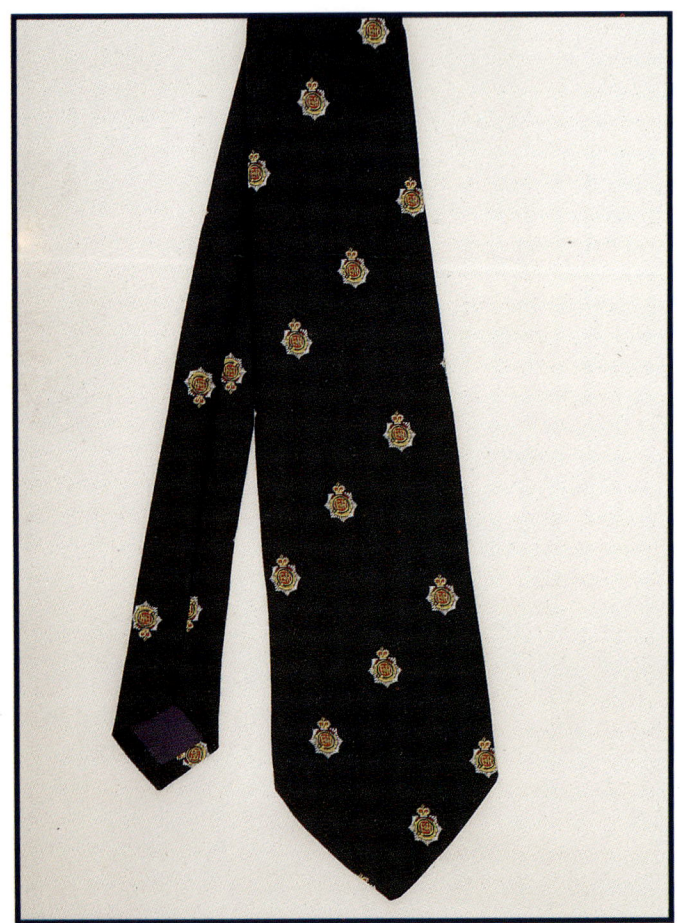

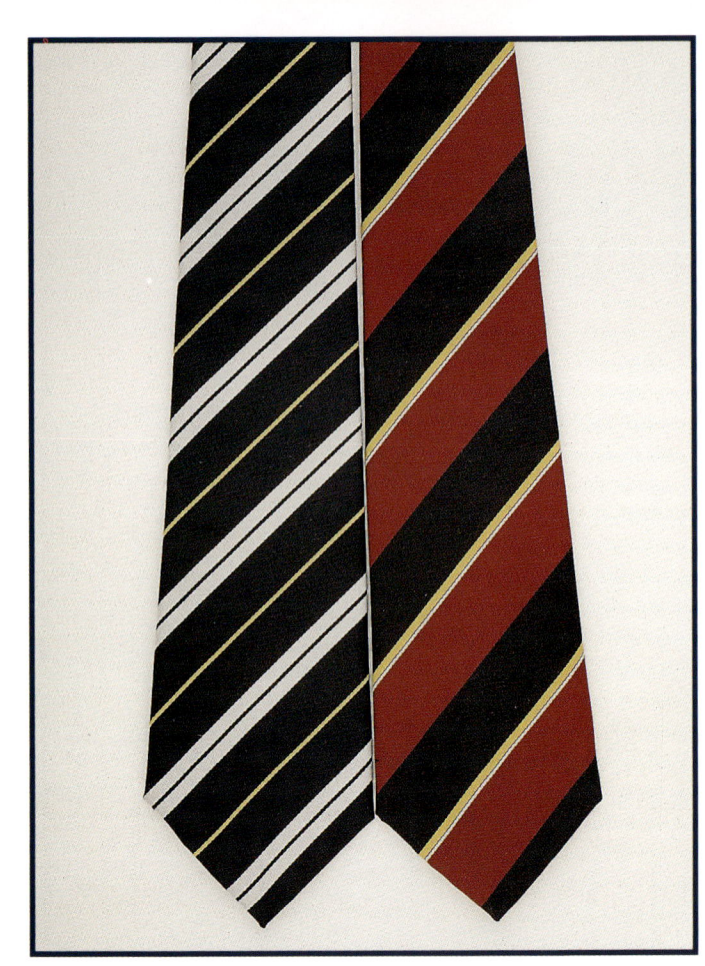

Royal Army Service Corps, crest

Royal Army Service Corps, stripe; Royal Army Pay Corps

Royal Artillery; Royal Army Veterinary Corps

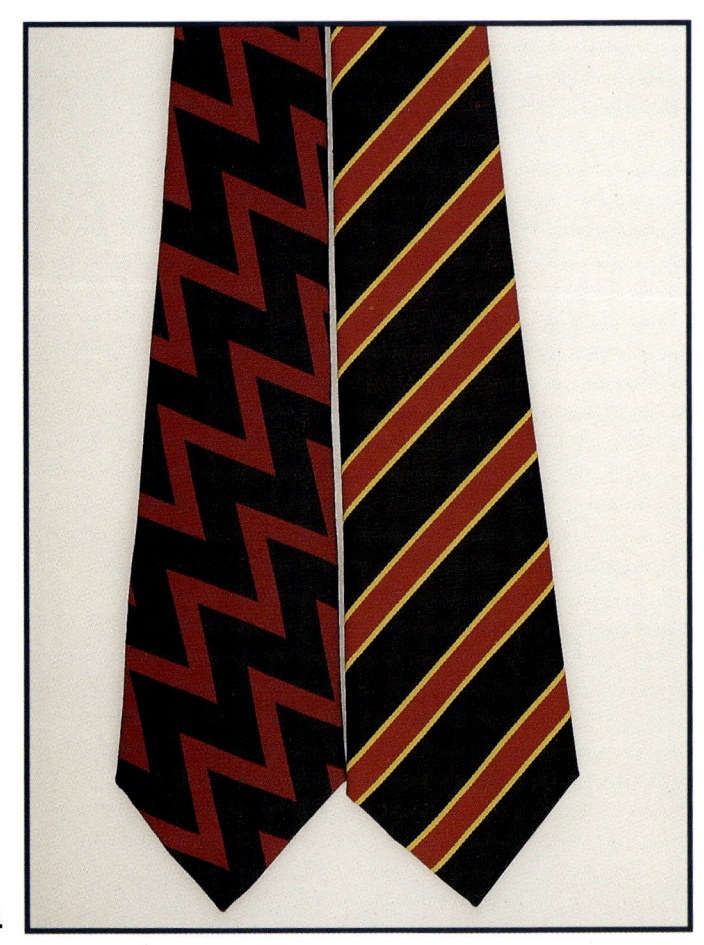

Royal Artillery, gold motifs
on maroon and navy

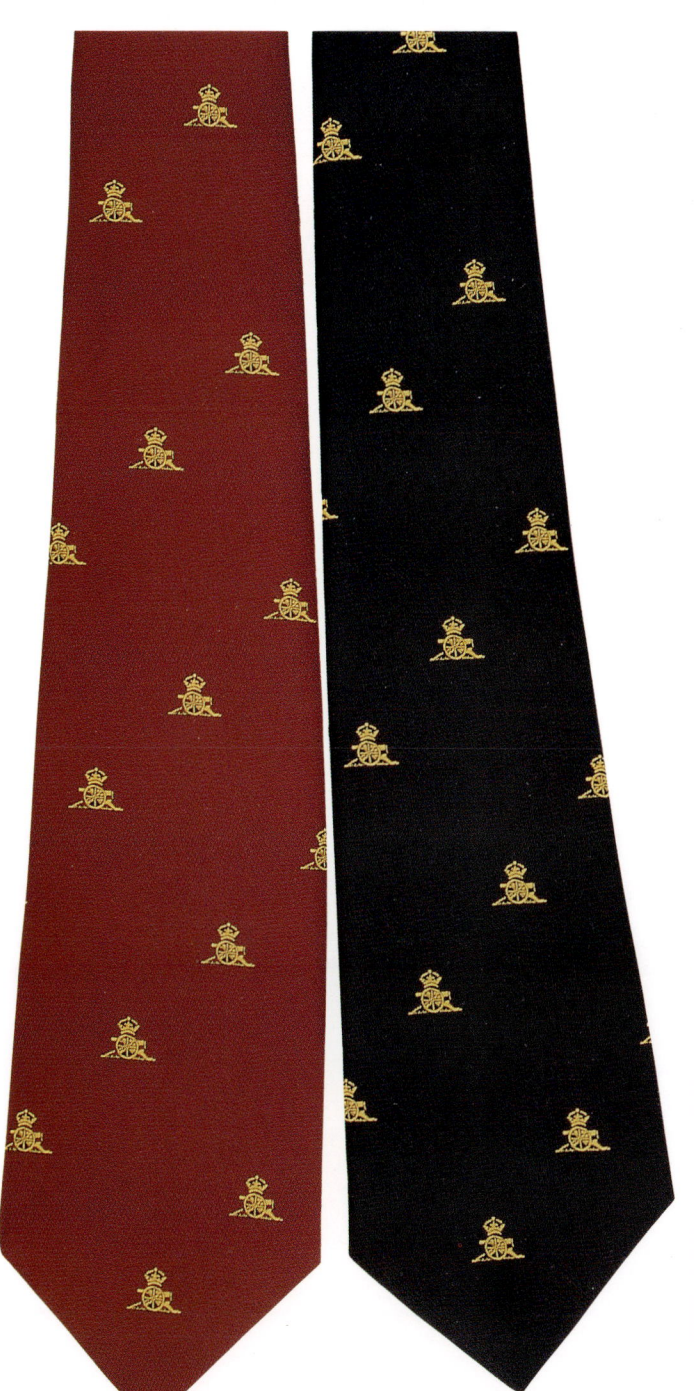

Royal Artillery, silver
motifs on maroon;
Royal Corps of Signals

55

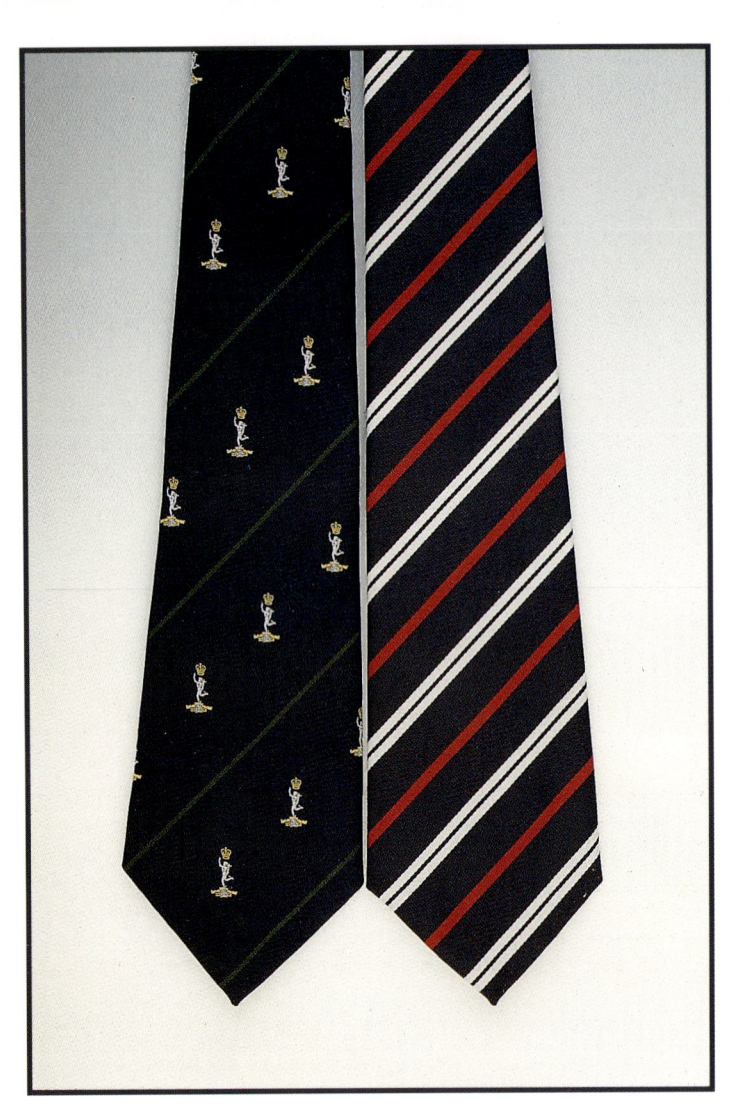

Royal Corps of Signals; Royal Corps of Transport

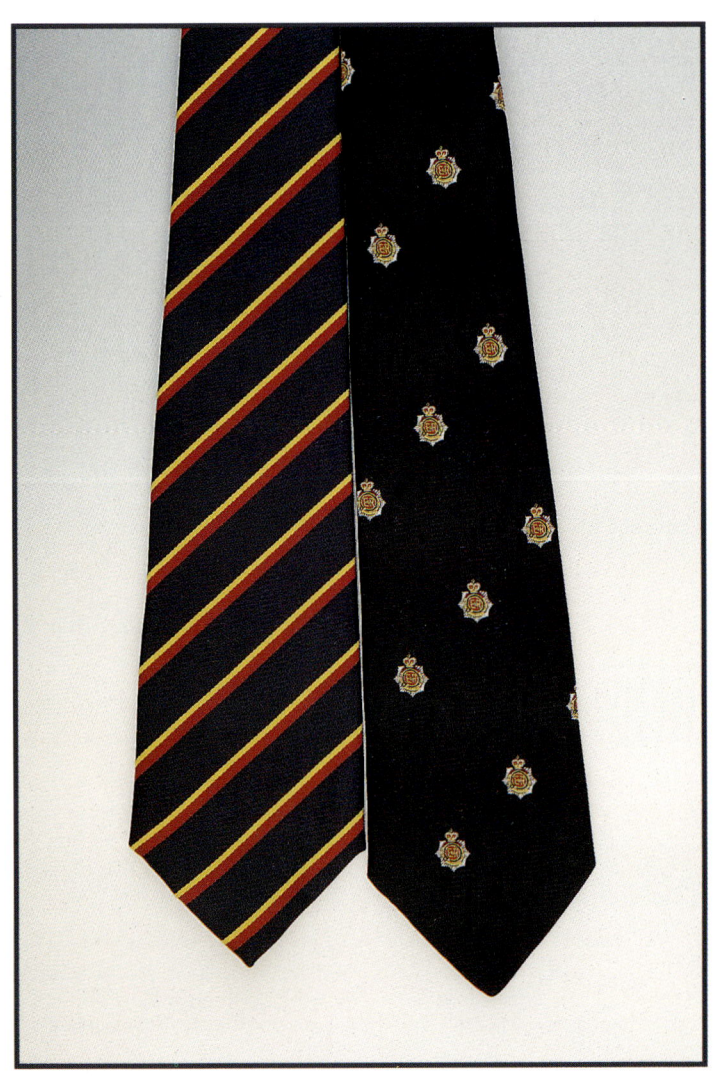

Royal Electrical and Mechanical Engineers, stripes; Royal Corps of Transport

56

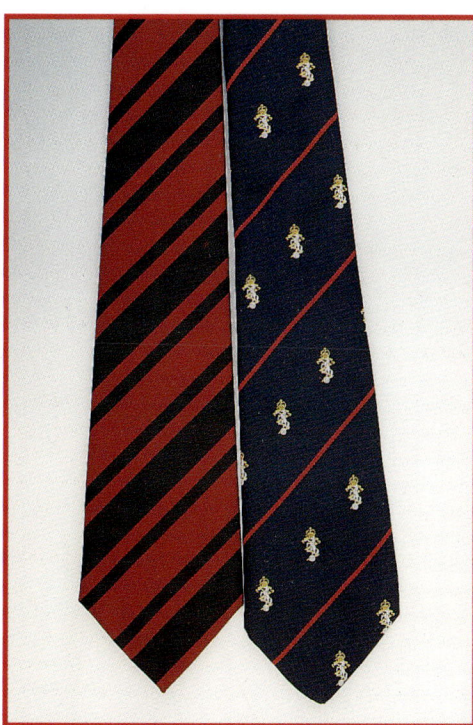

Royal Engineers; Royal
Electrical and Mechanical
Engineers, crest

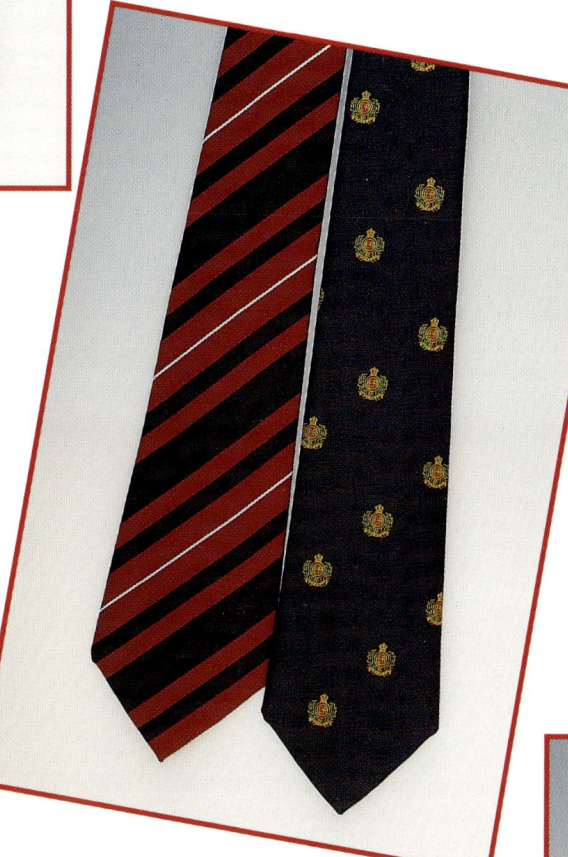

Royal Engineers
(Territorials); Royal
Engineers, crest

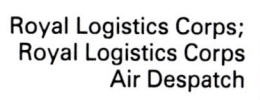

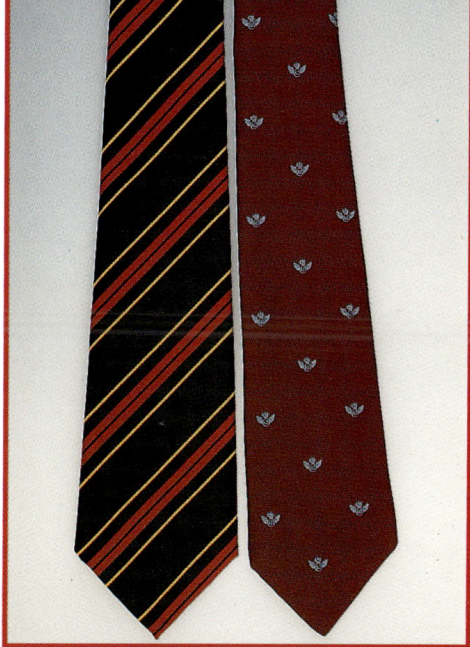

Royal Logistics Corps;
Royal Logistics Corps
Air Despatch

57

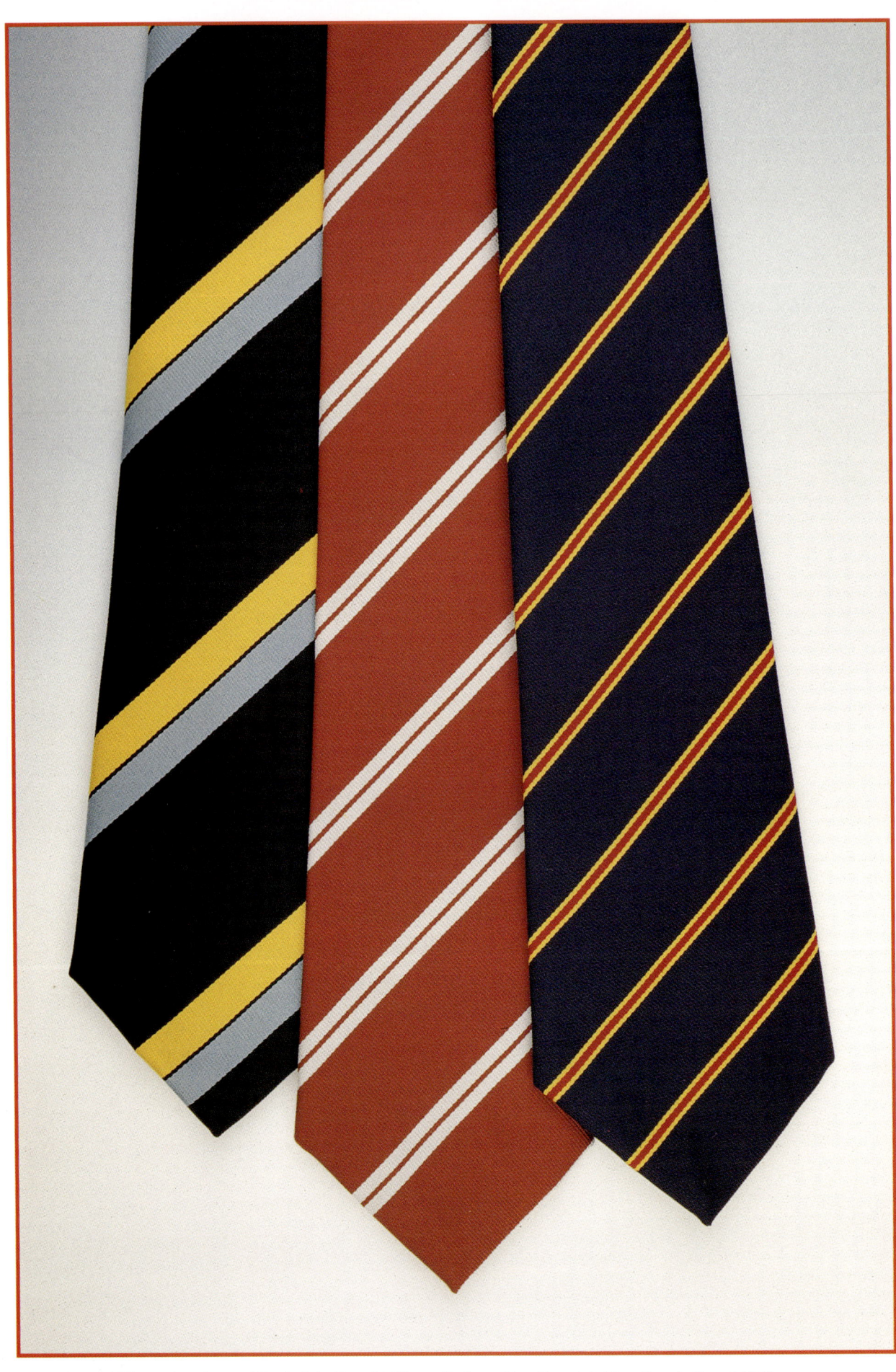

Royal Military Academy, Woolwich; Royal Military College Sandhurst (old pattern); Royal Military Academy, Sandhurst

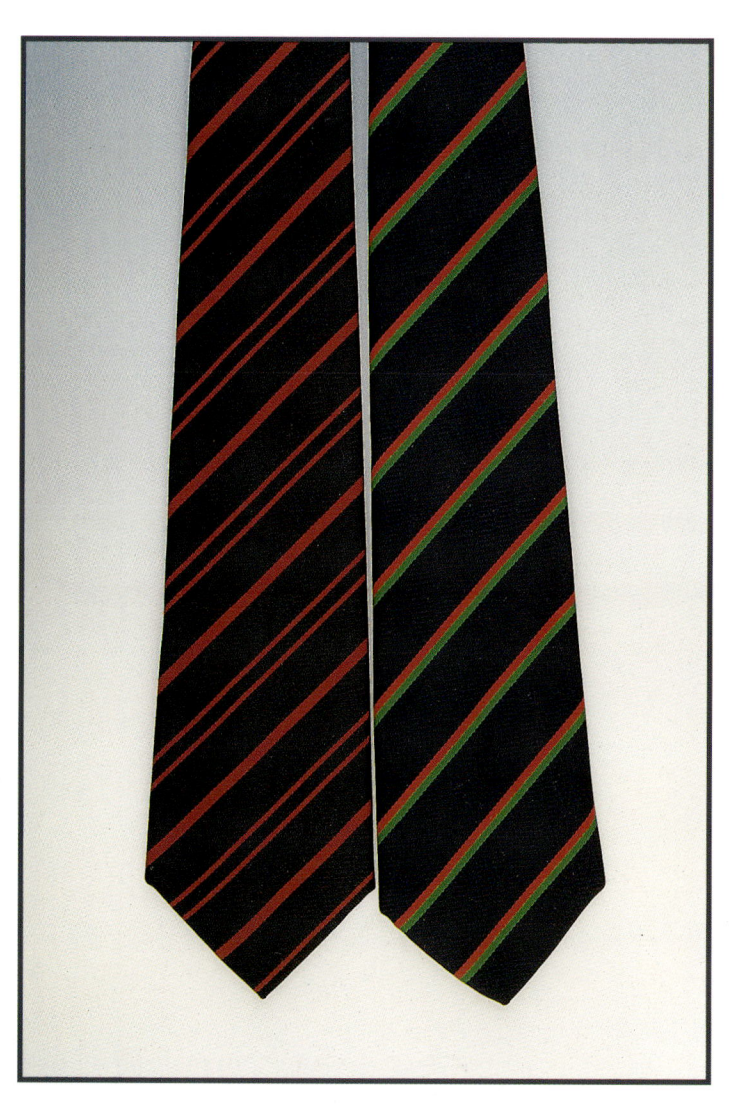

Royal Military Police; Royal Pioneer Corps

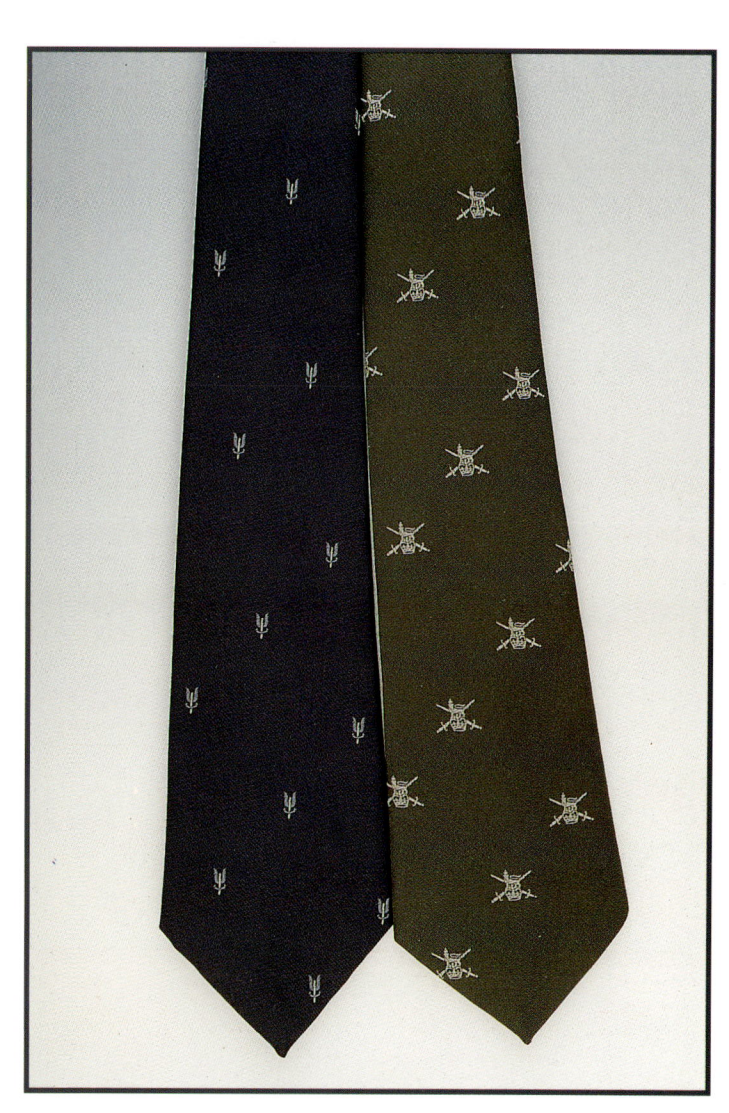

Special Air Service; Territorial Army

59

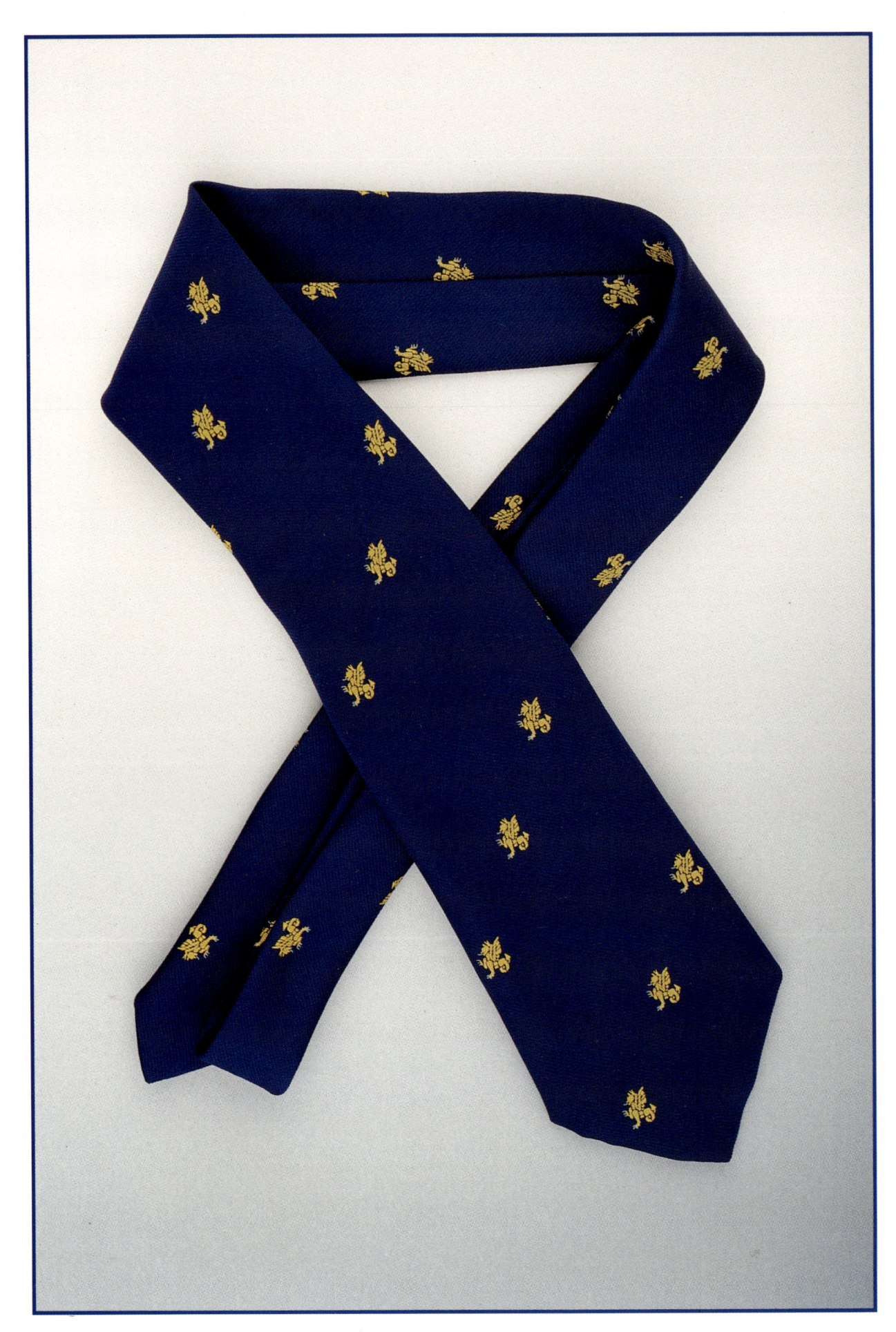

43rd Wessex Division

Naval

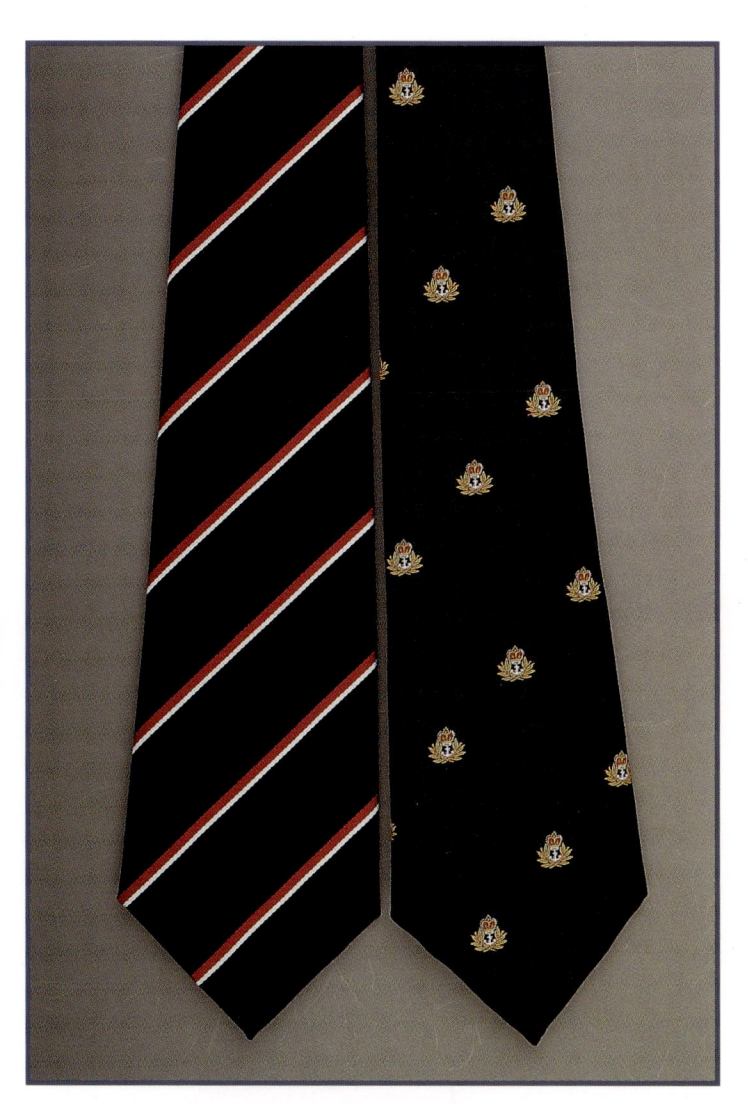

Royal Navy, stripe and cap-badge motif

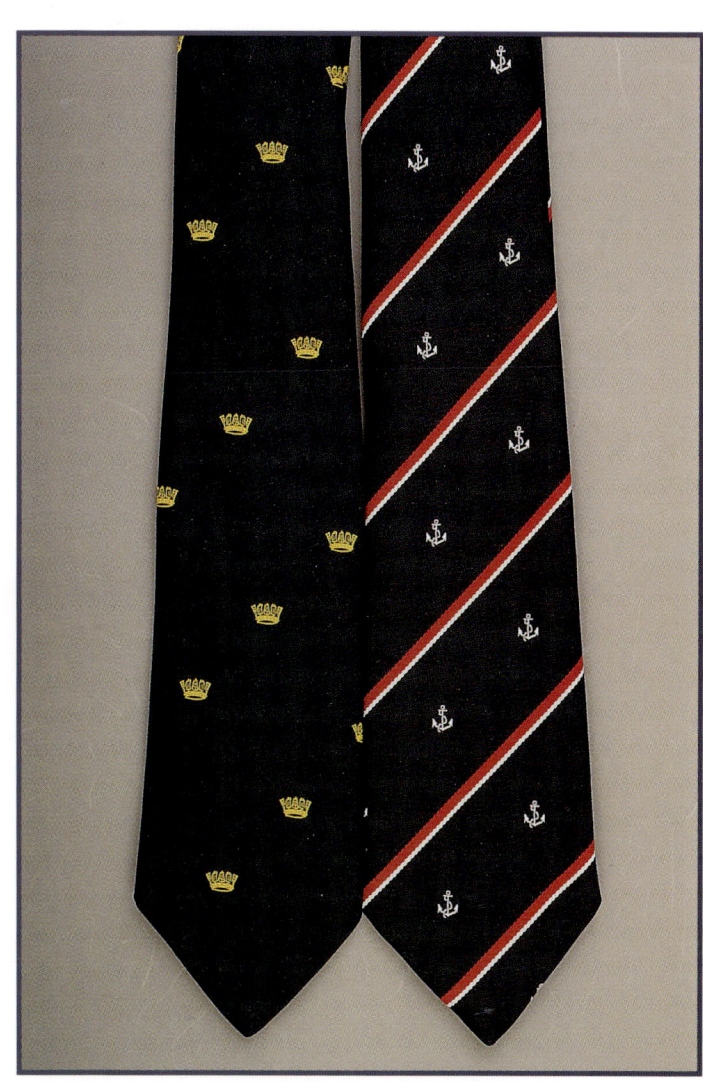

Royal Navy, gold crown and stripe and anchor

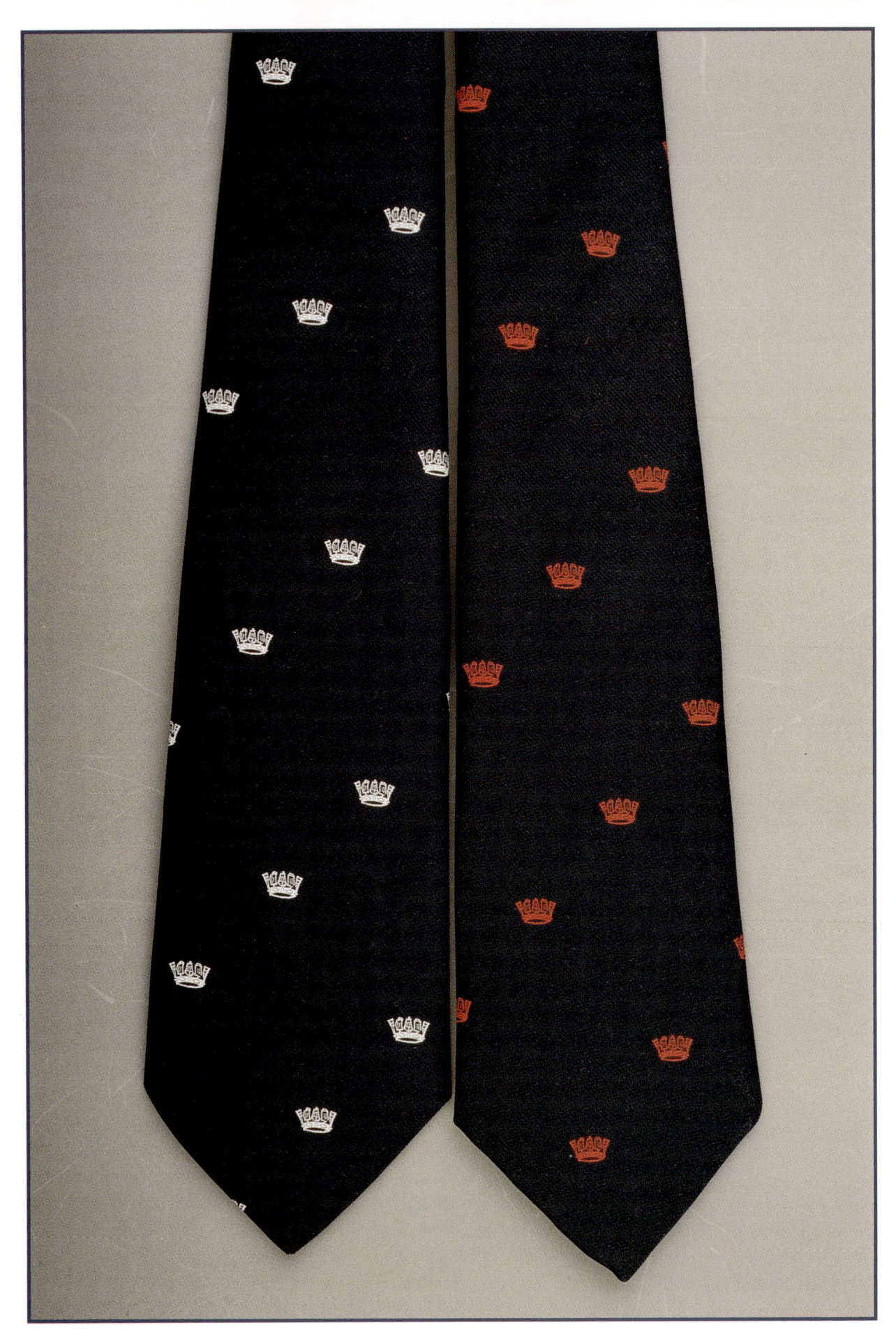

Royal Navy Devonport; Royal Navy Portsmouth

62

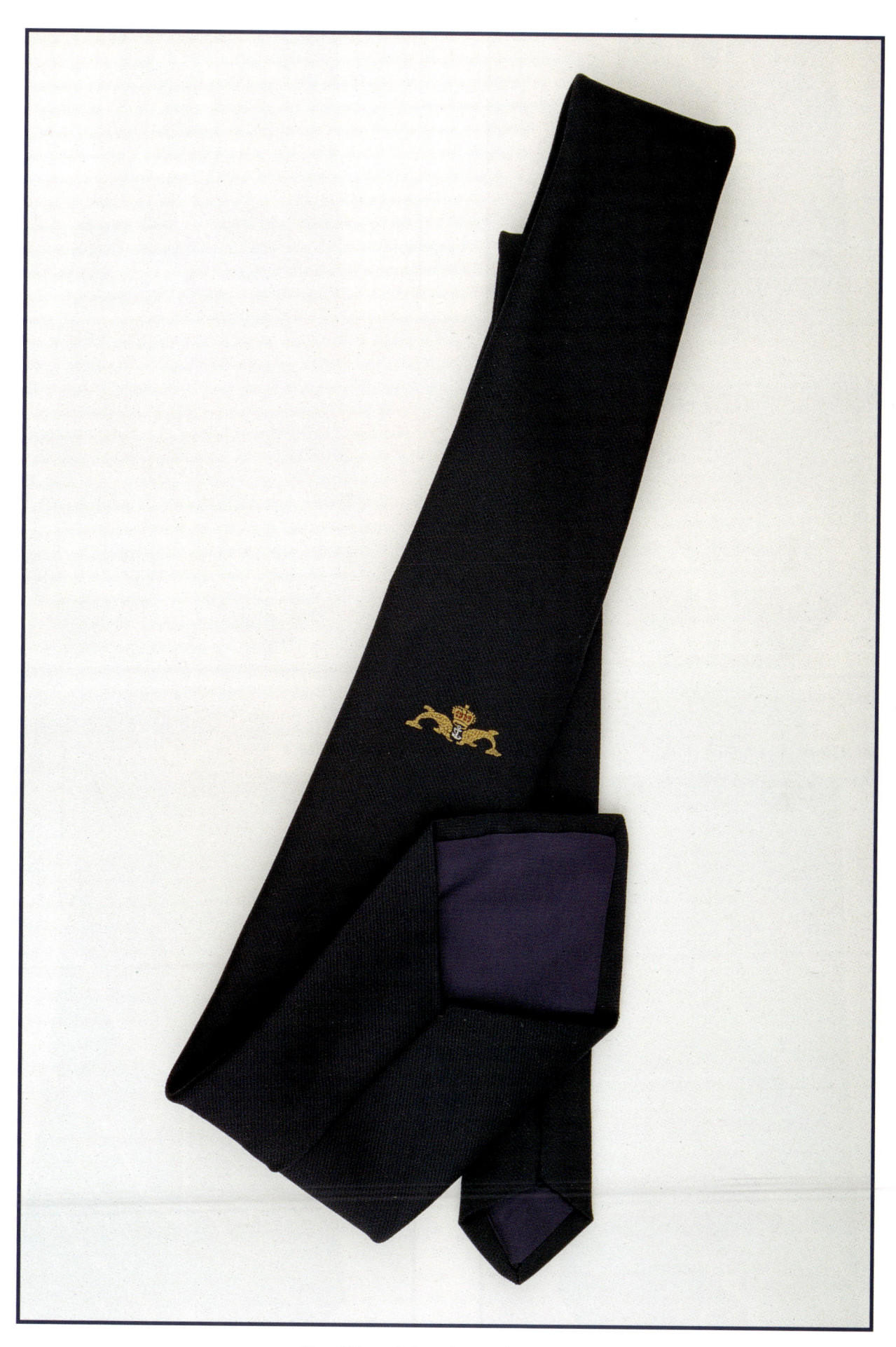

Royal Navy Submariners, single motif

Royal Marines

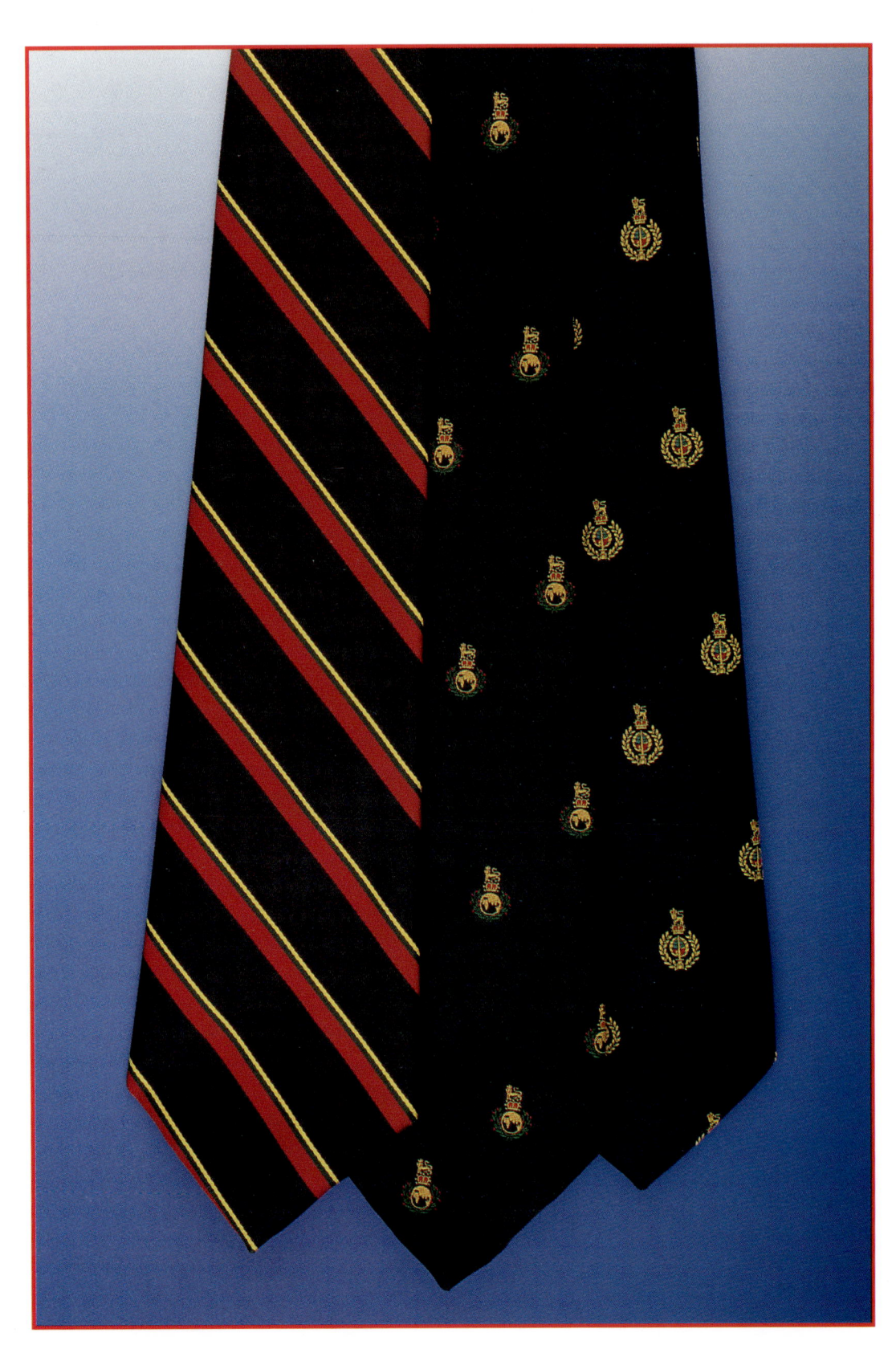

Royal Marines, stripe and crest; Royal Marines Commando

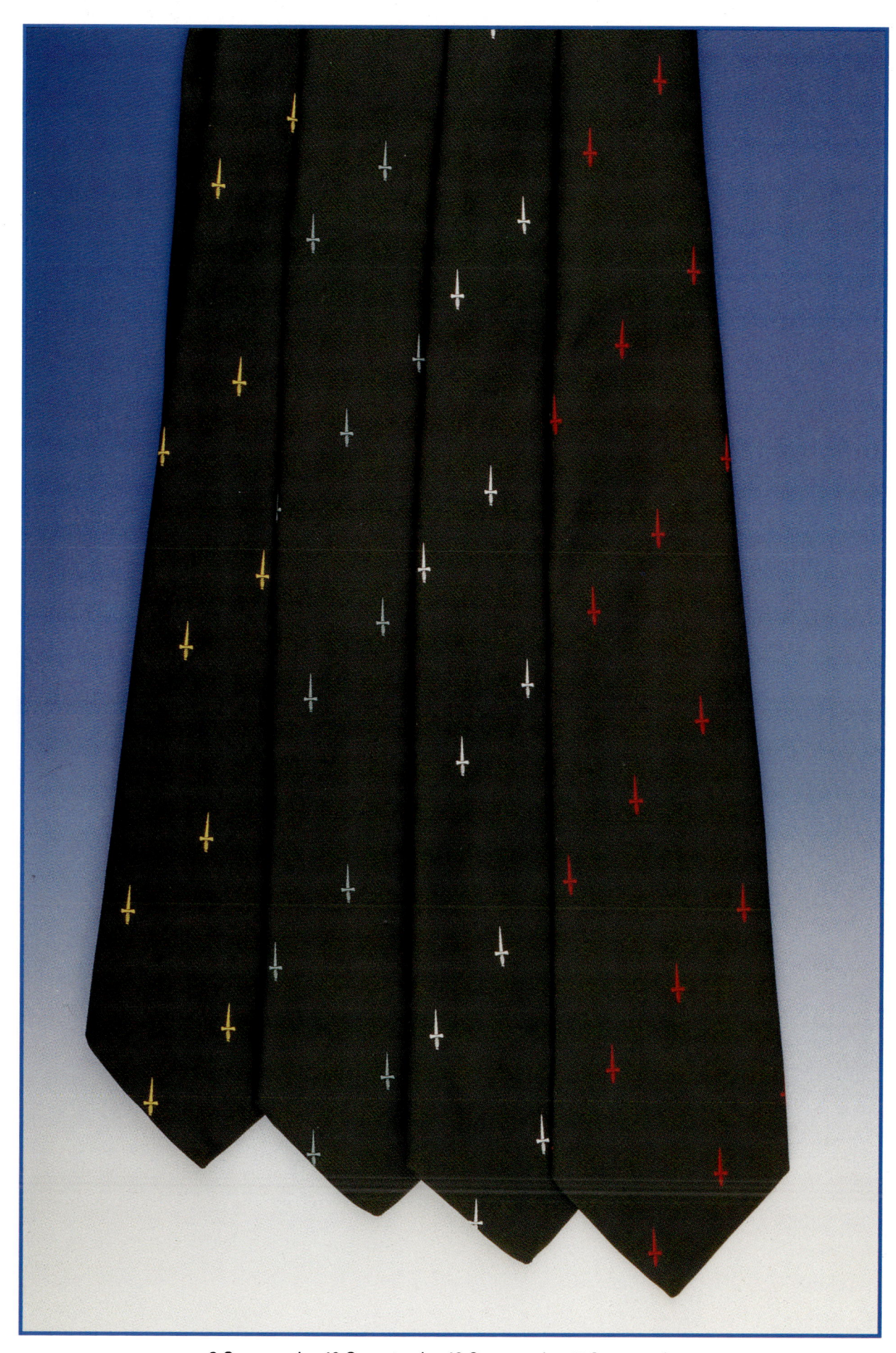

3 Commando; 40 Commando; 42 Commando; 45 Commando

Air Force

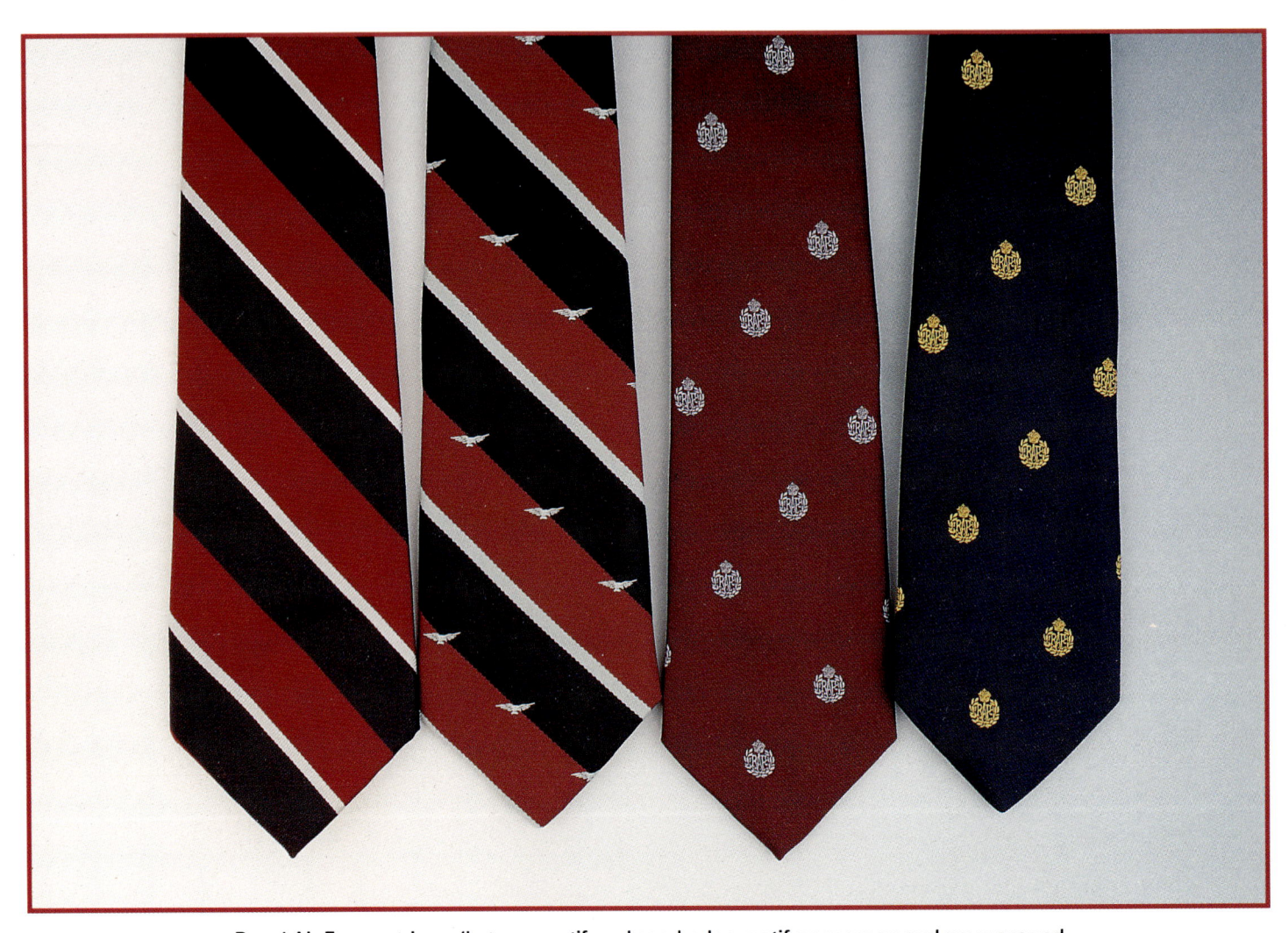

Royal Air Force, stripe, albatross motif, and cap-badge motif on maroon and navy ground

Royal Flying Corps

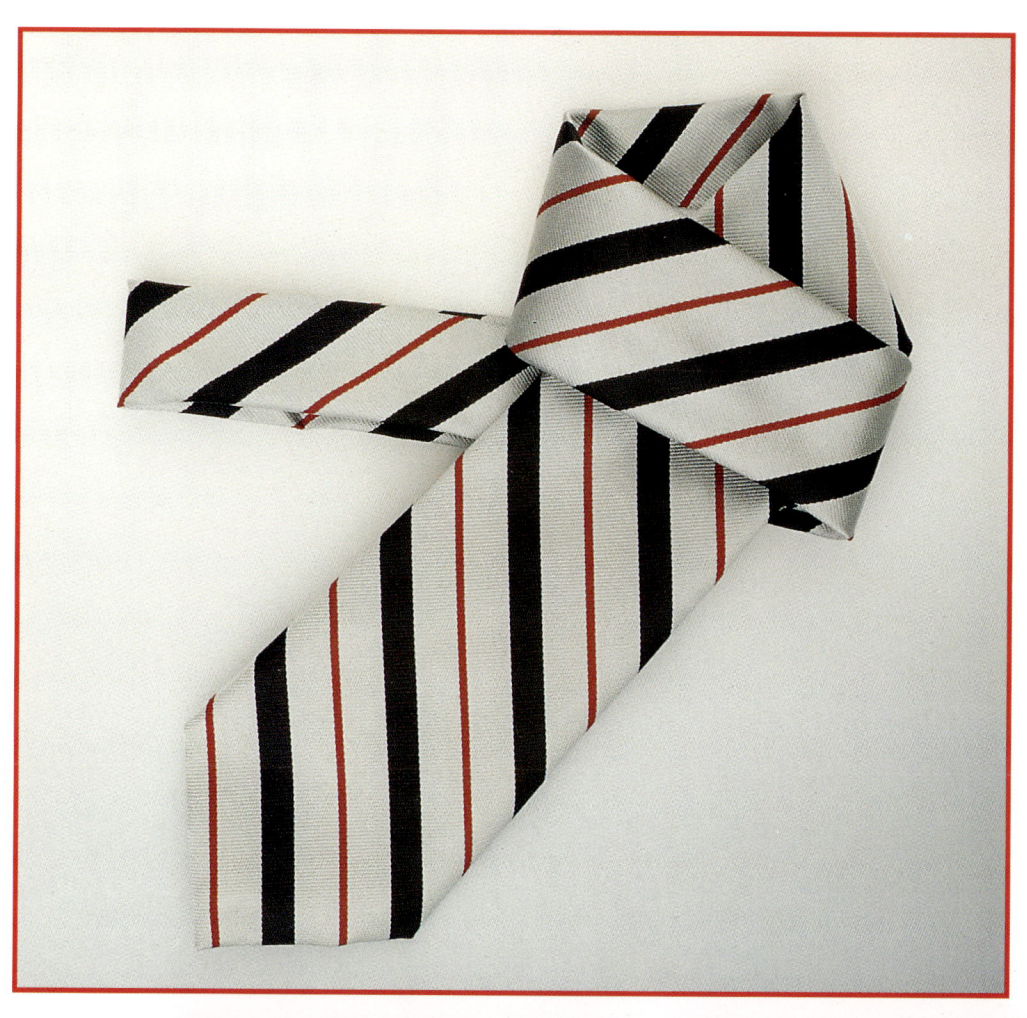

R.A.F. Pilot; R.A.F. Bomb-aimer; R.A.F. Navigator; R.A.F. Observer

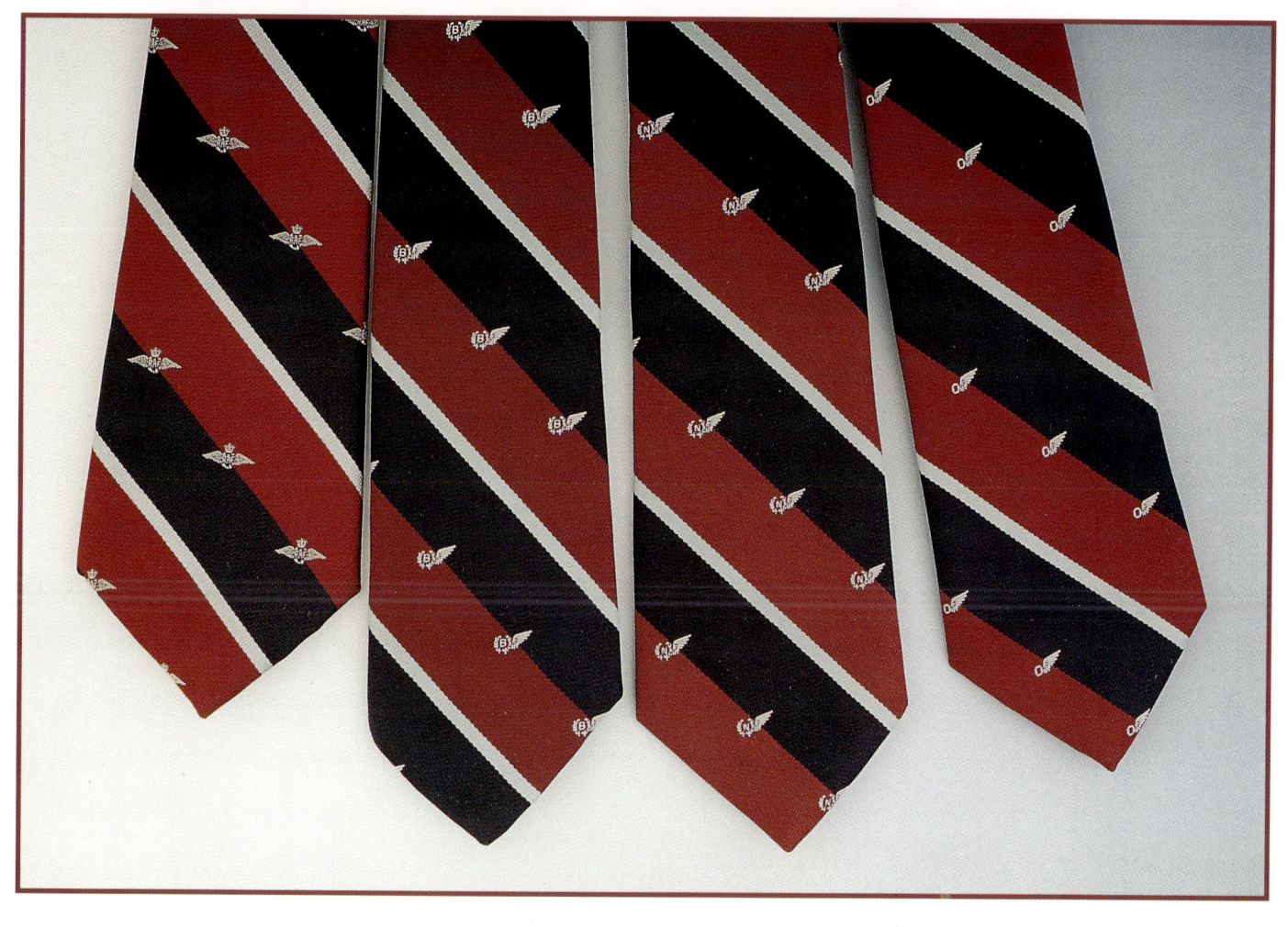

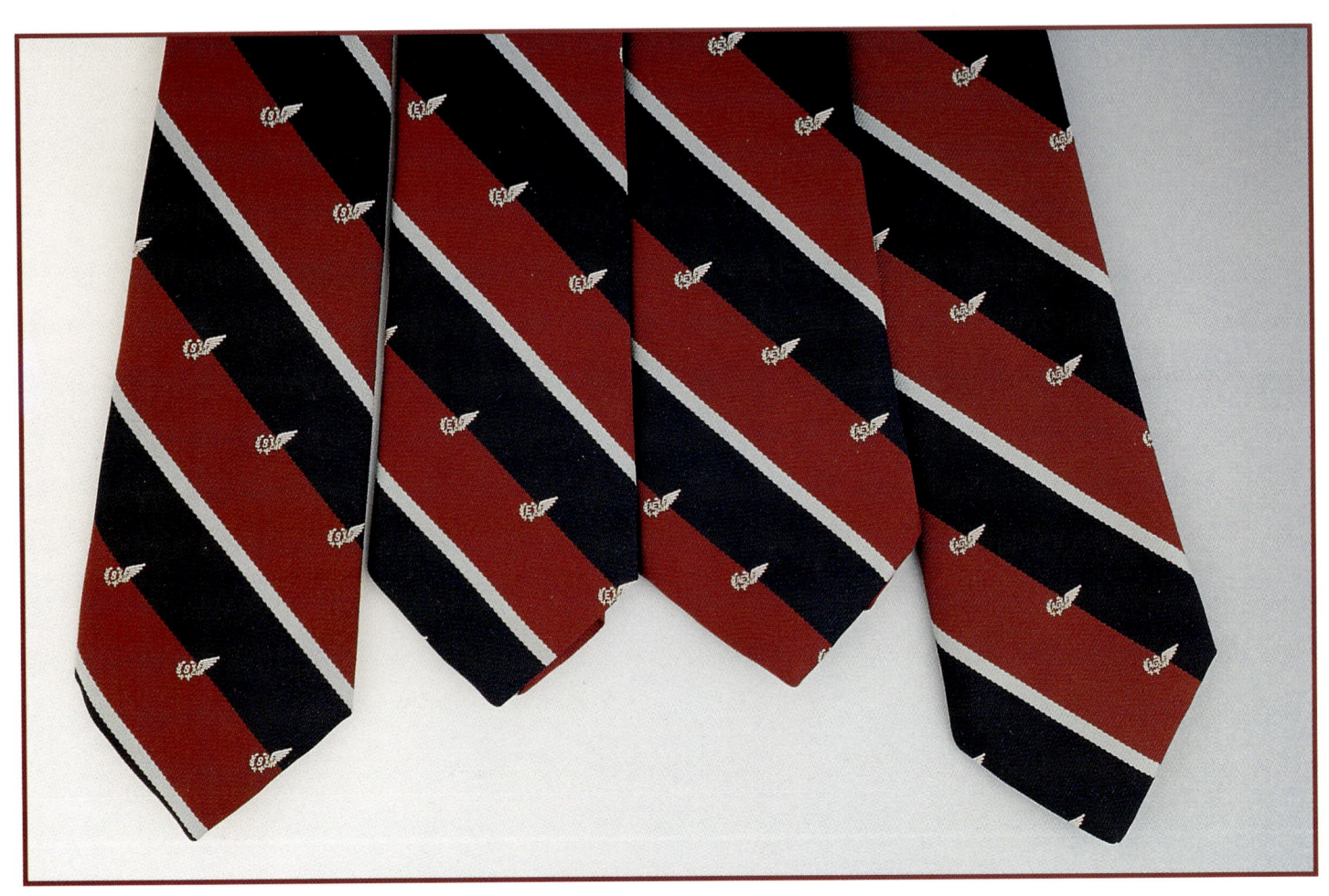

R.A.F. Signaller; R.A.F. Engineer; R.A.F. Air Electronics; R.A.F. Air Gunner

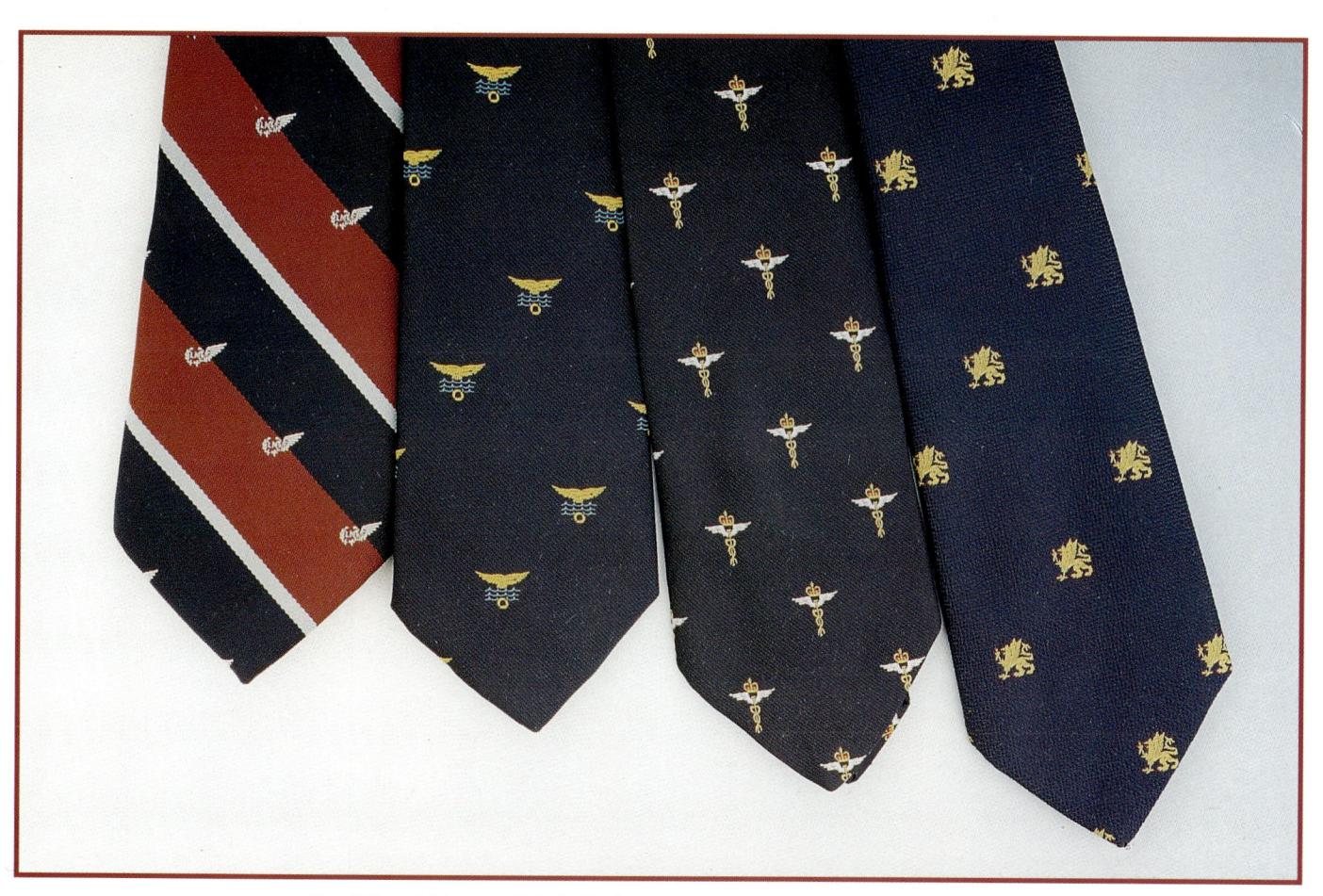

R.A.F. Load Master; R.A.F. Air-Sea Rescue; R.A.F. Medical; R.A.F. Police
R.A.F. Regiment striped and crest; R.A.F. Warrant Officer; Air Training Corps

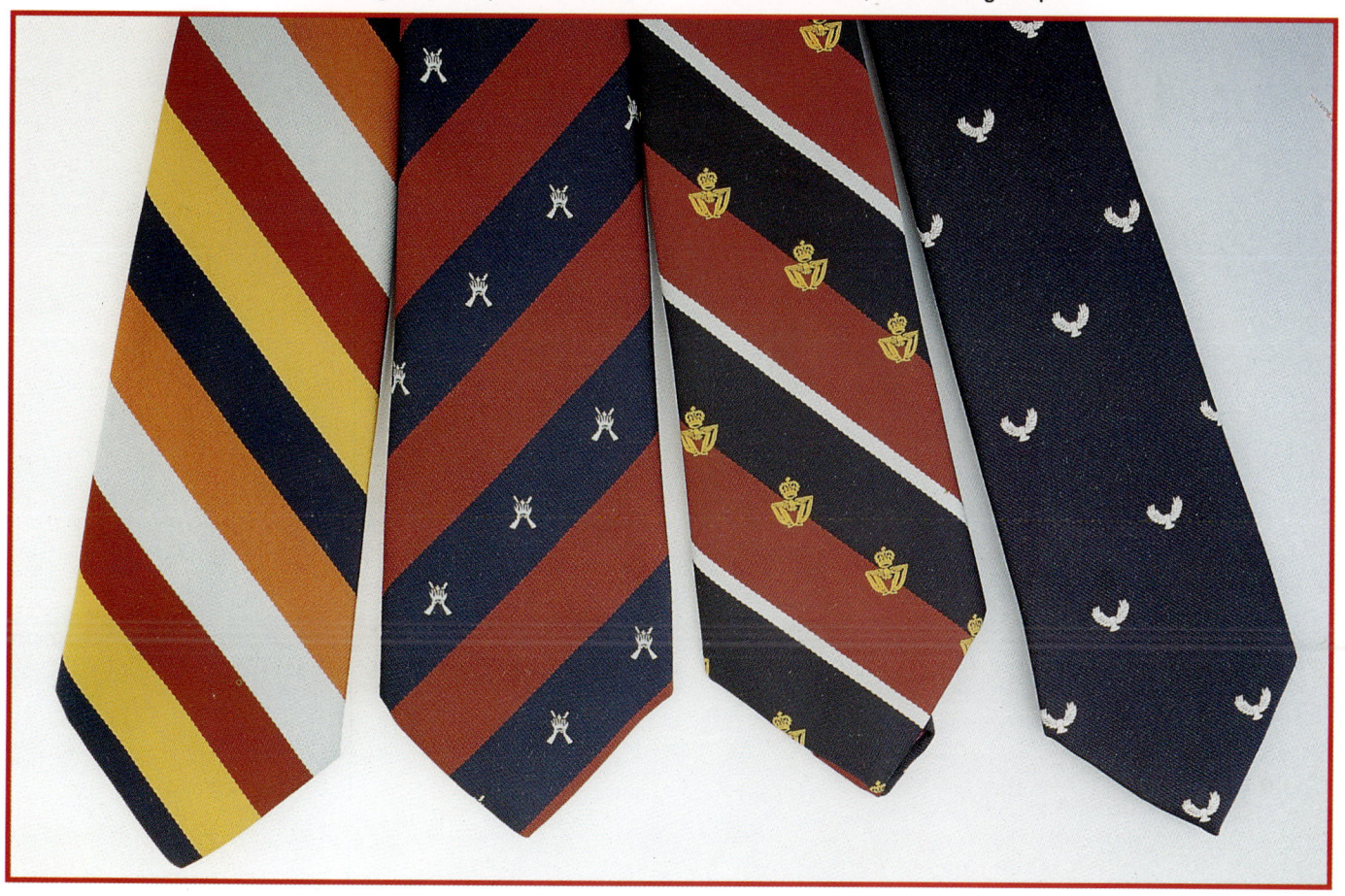

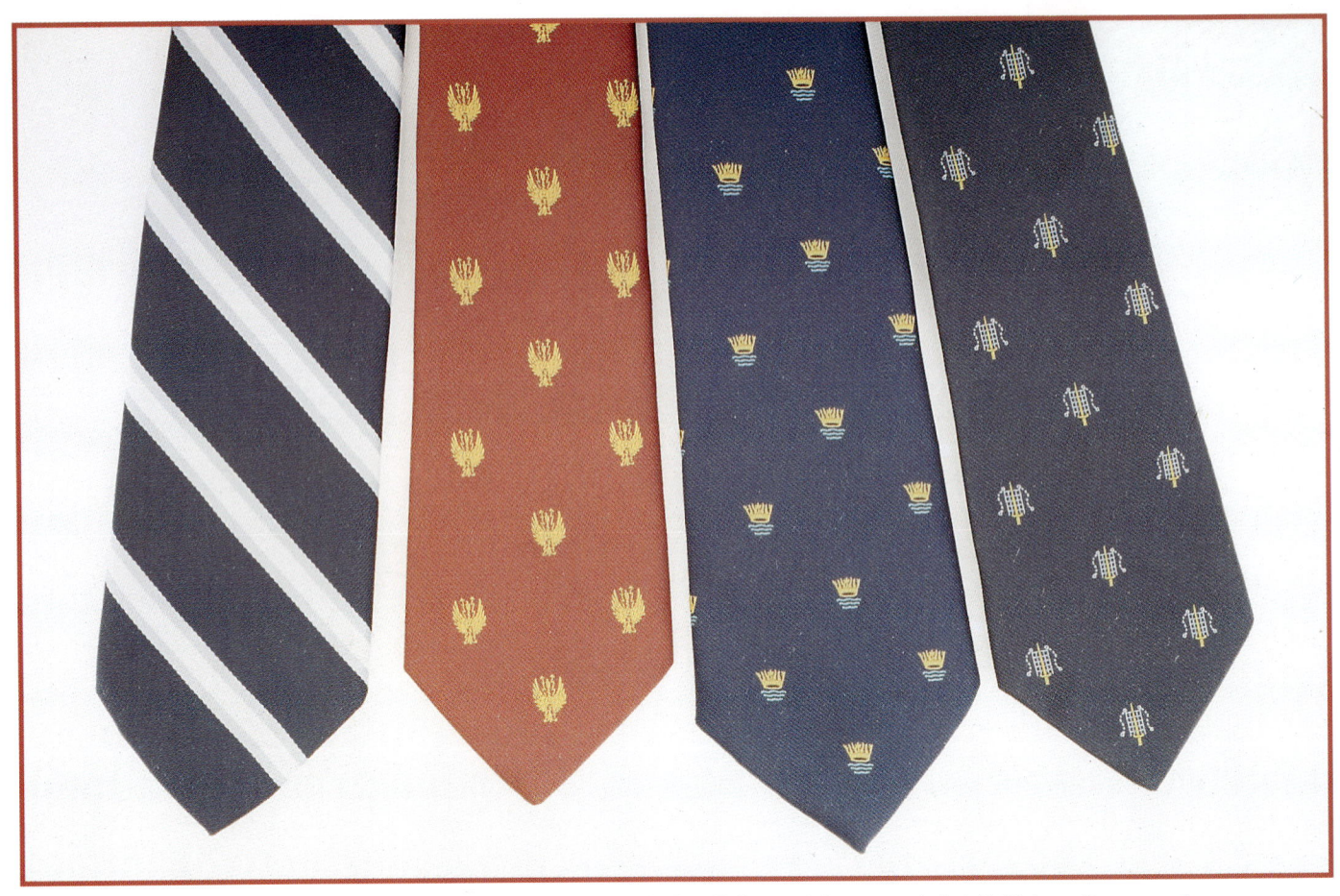

Royal Observer Corps; R.A.F. Bomber Command; R.A.F. Coastal Command; R.A.F. Fighter Command

R.A.F. Desert Air Force; R.A.F. Volunteer Reserve; Royal Air Force Association; Royal Canadian Air Force Pilot; R.A.F. Maintenance Command

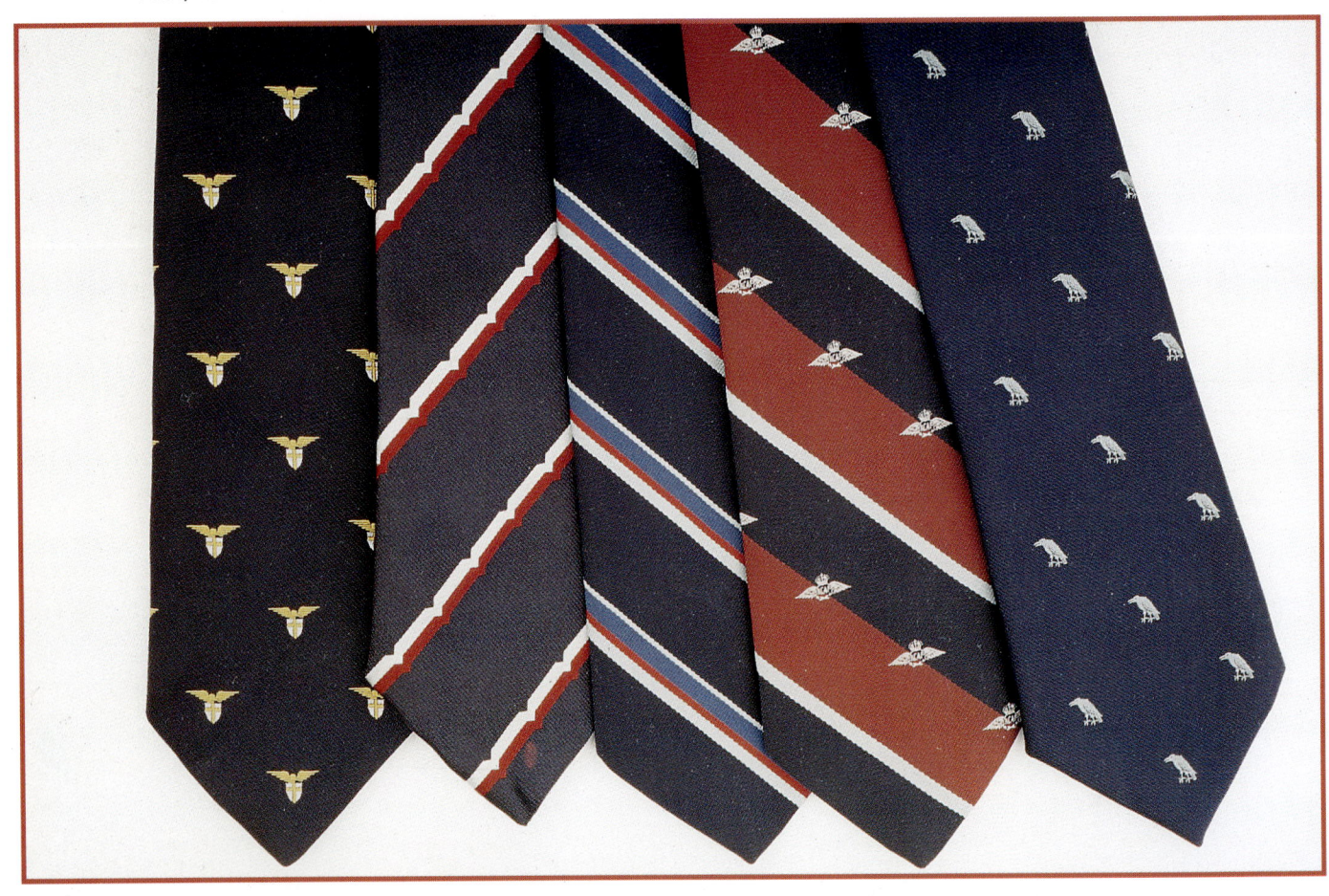

Universities

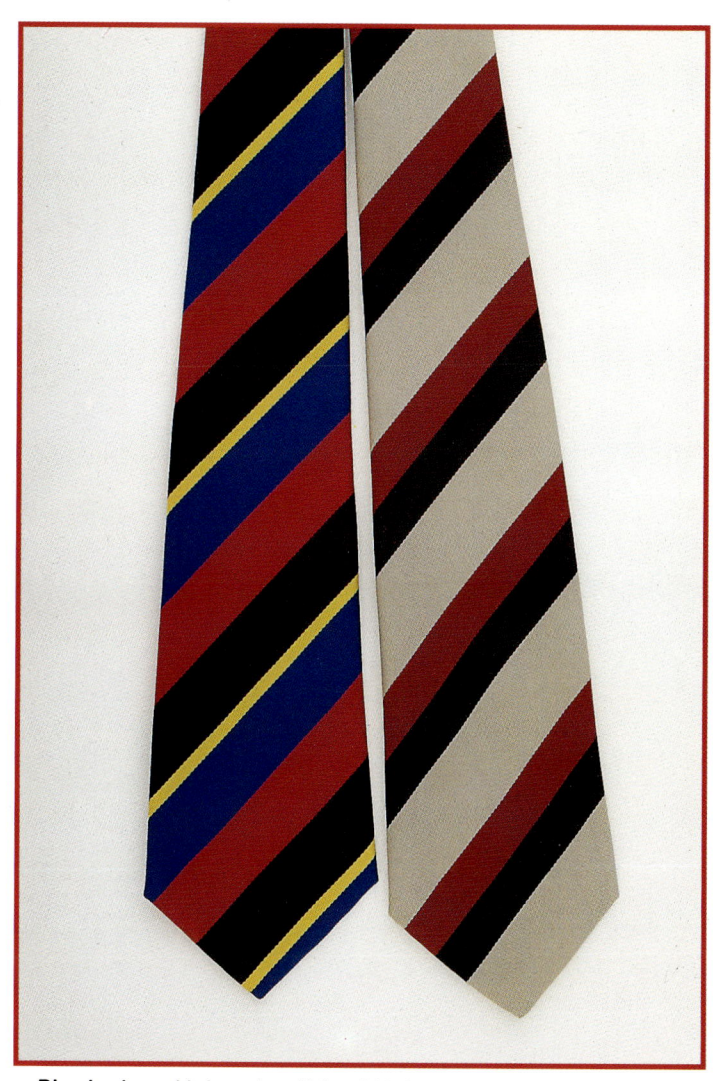

Birmingham University; Bristol University

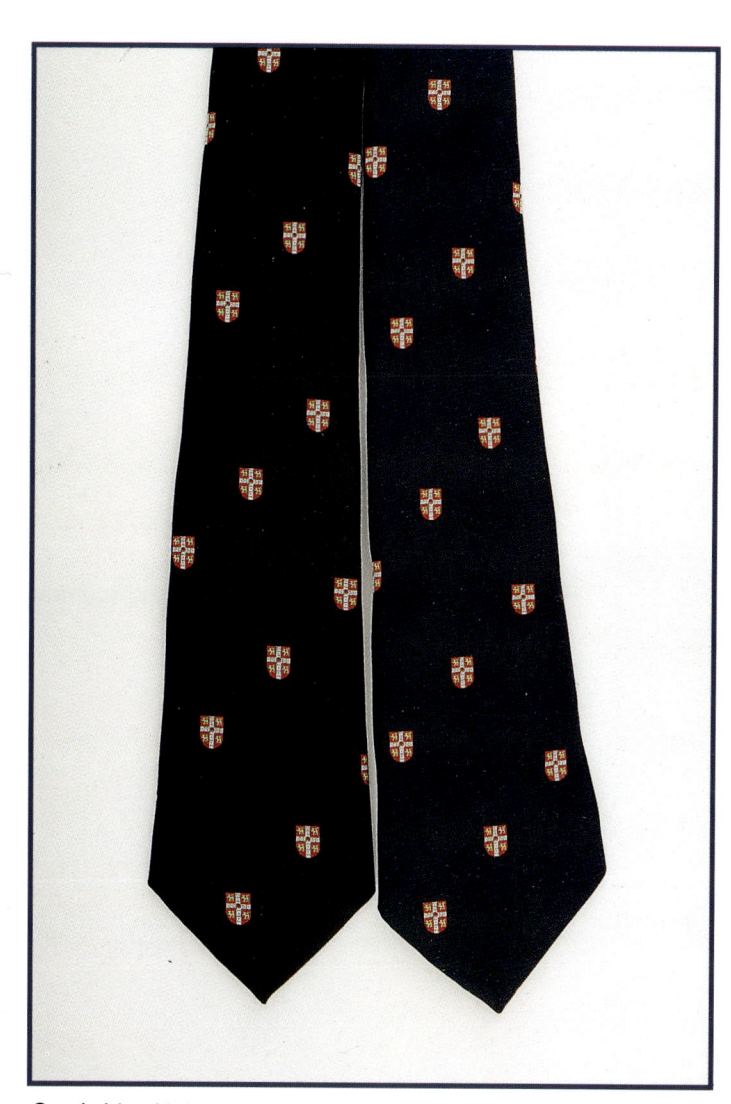

Cambridge University, black and navy grounds

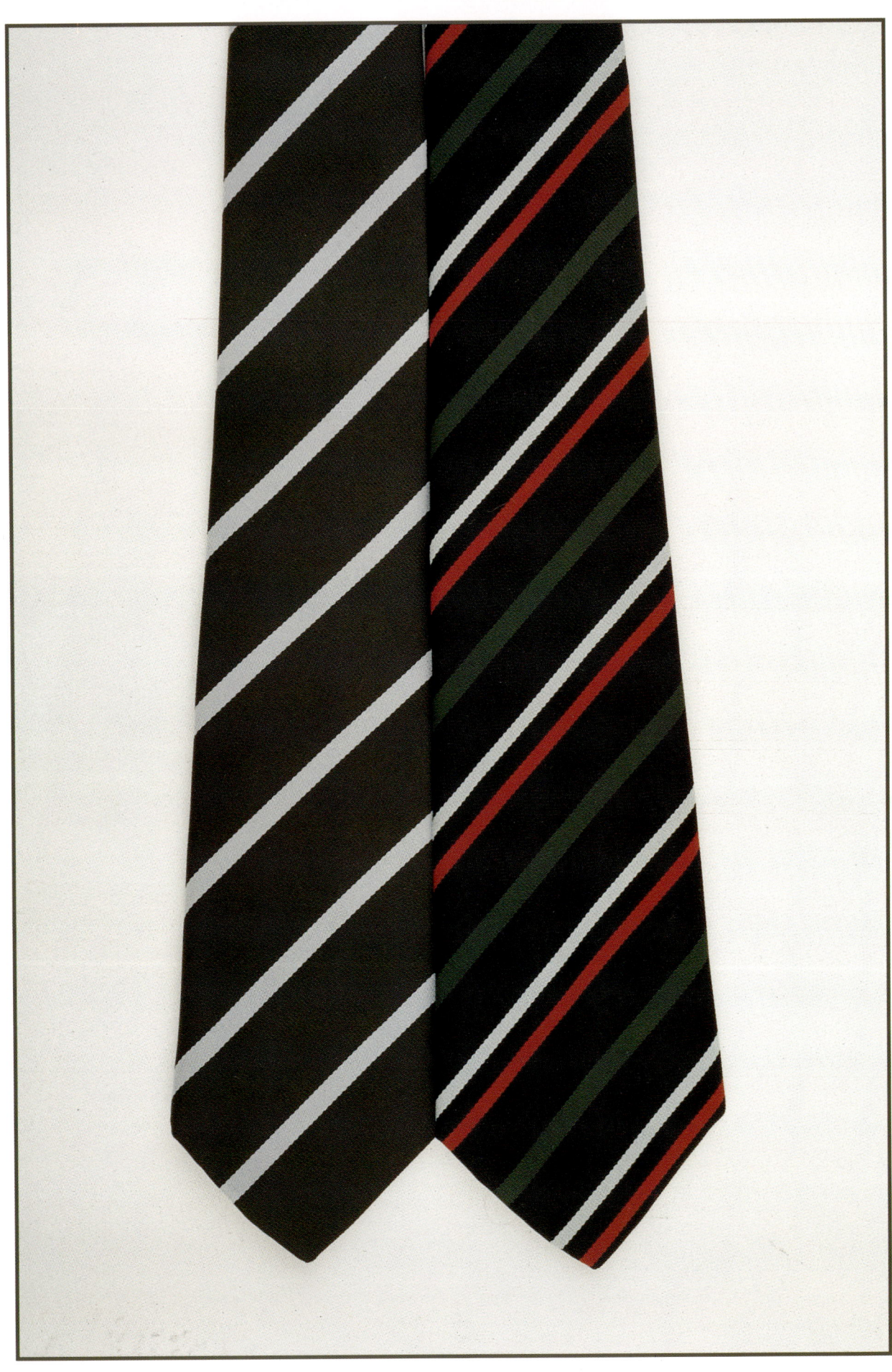

Cardiff University; Trinity College Dublin

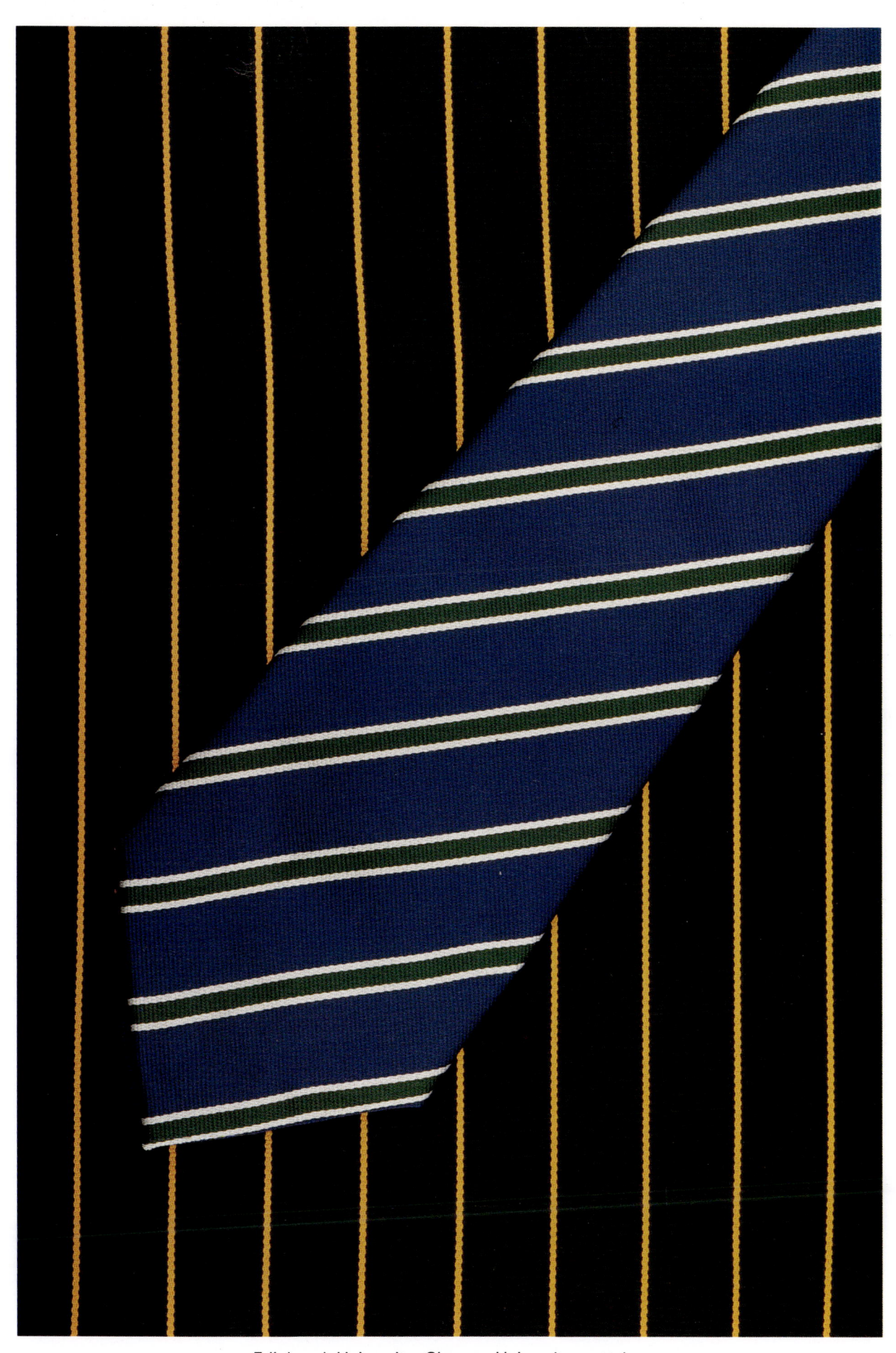

Edinburgh University; Glasgow University, swatch

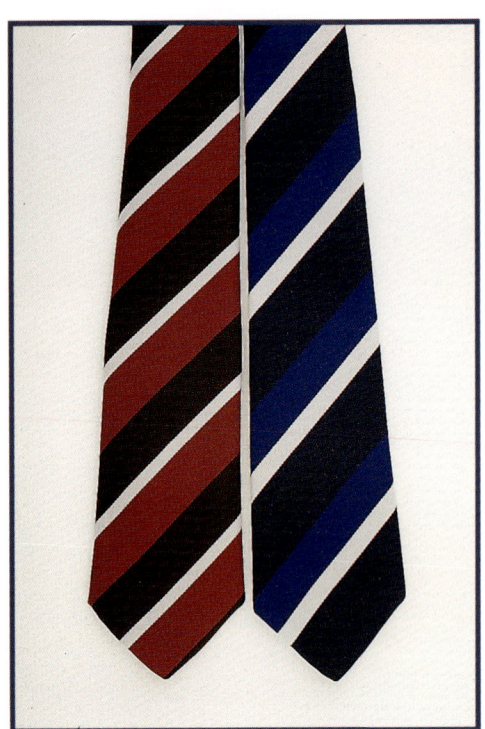

Leeds University;
Liverpool University

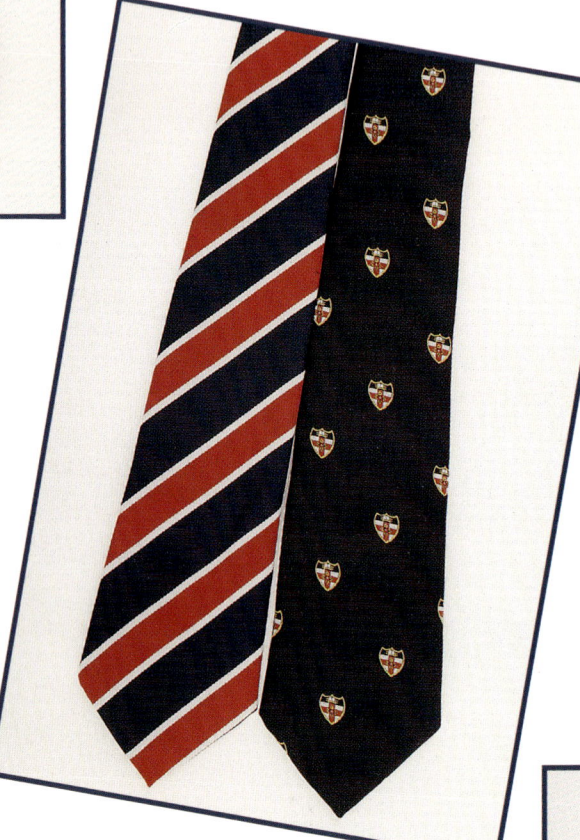

London University, stripe
and crest

Manchester University;
Nottingham University

76

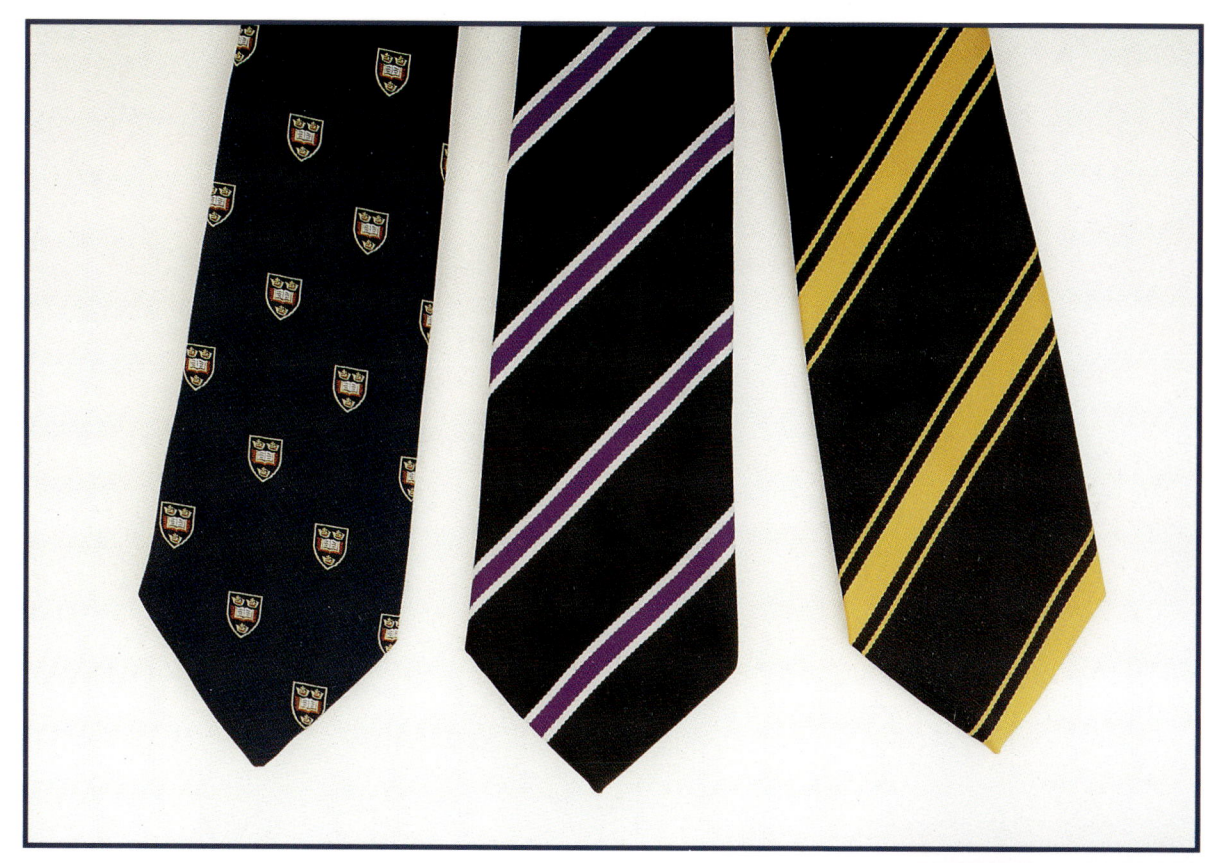

Oxford University; Reading University;
Sheffield University

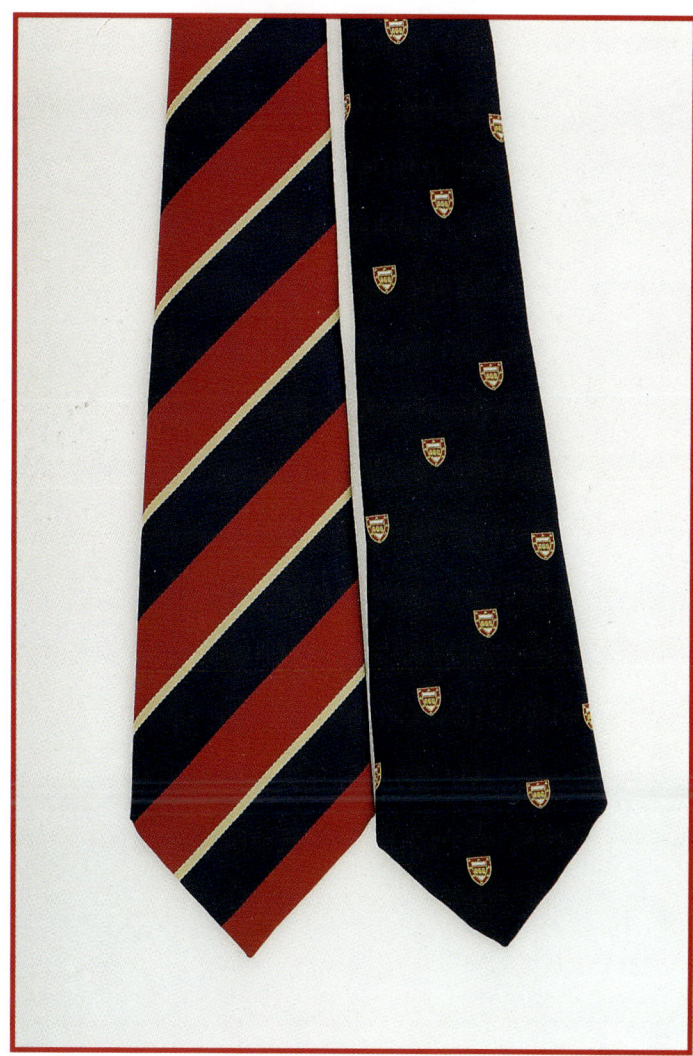

University of Wales,
stripe and crest

London Colleges, Medical Schools

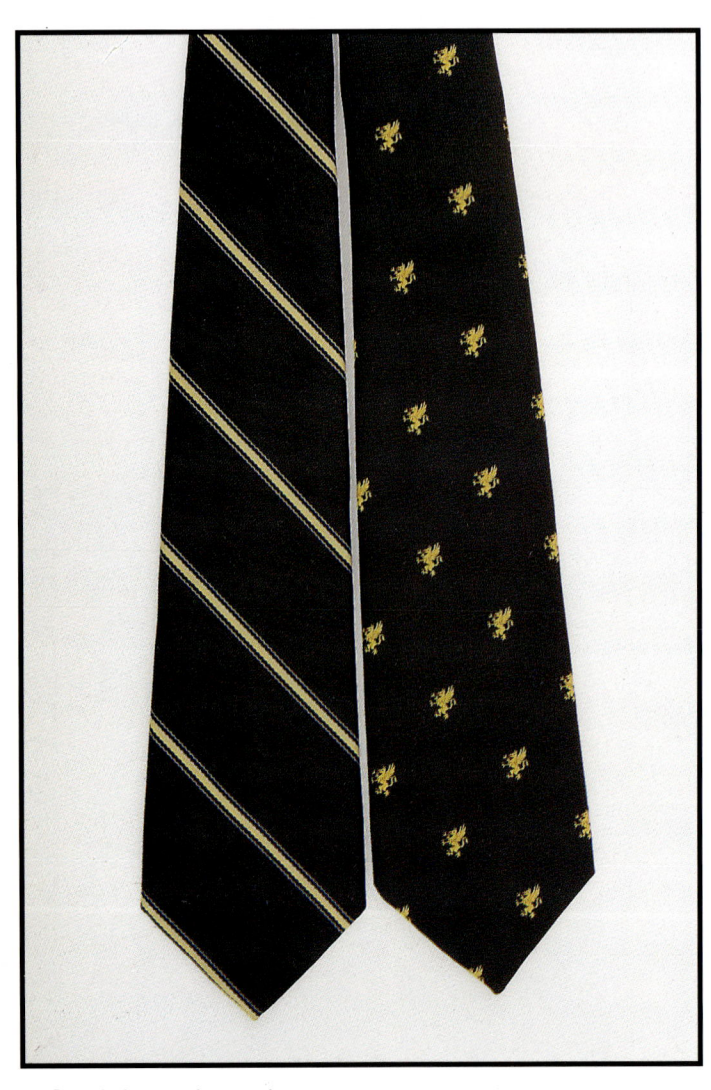

Gray's Inn, stripe and crest

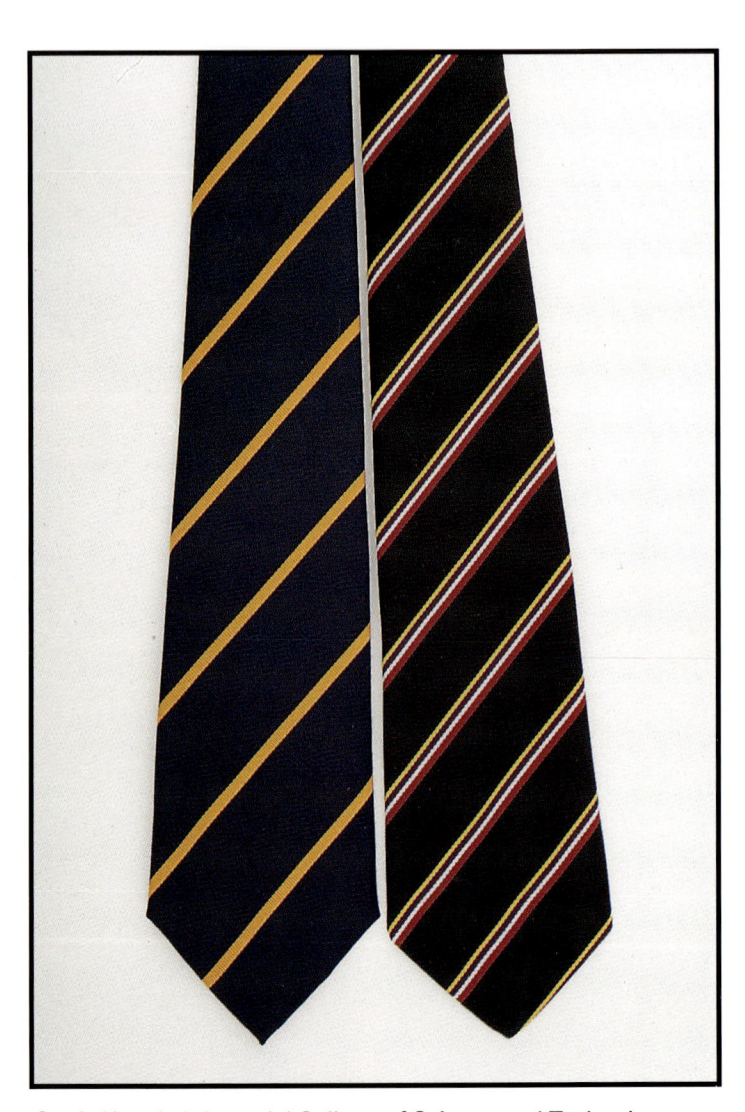

Guy's Hospital; Imperial College of Science and Technology

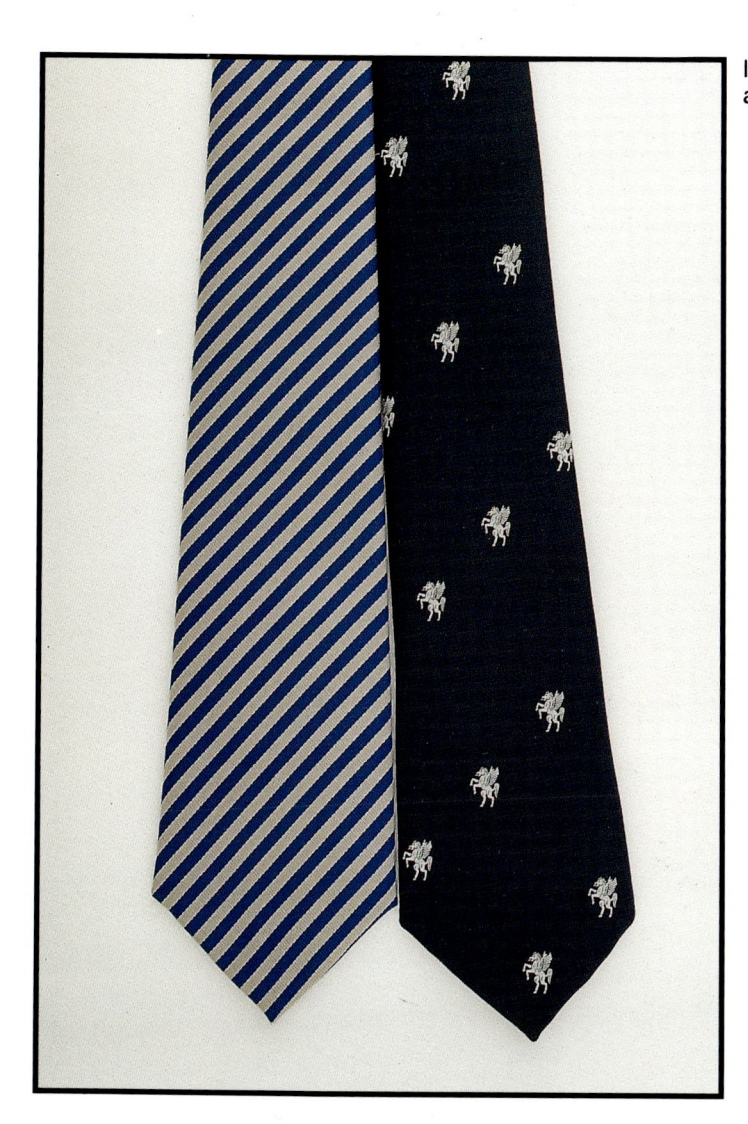

Inner Temple, stripe
and crest

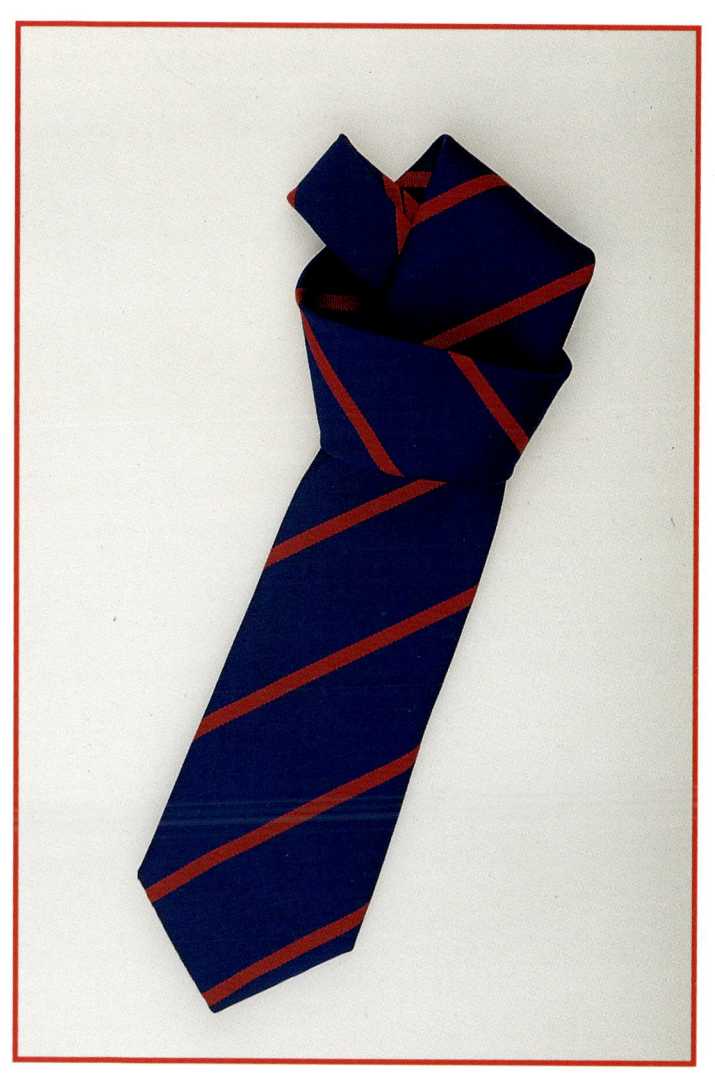

King's College

79

Lincoln's Inn, stripe and crest

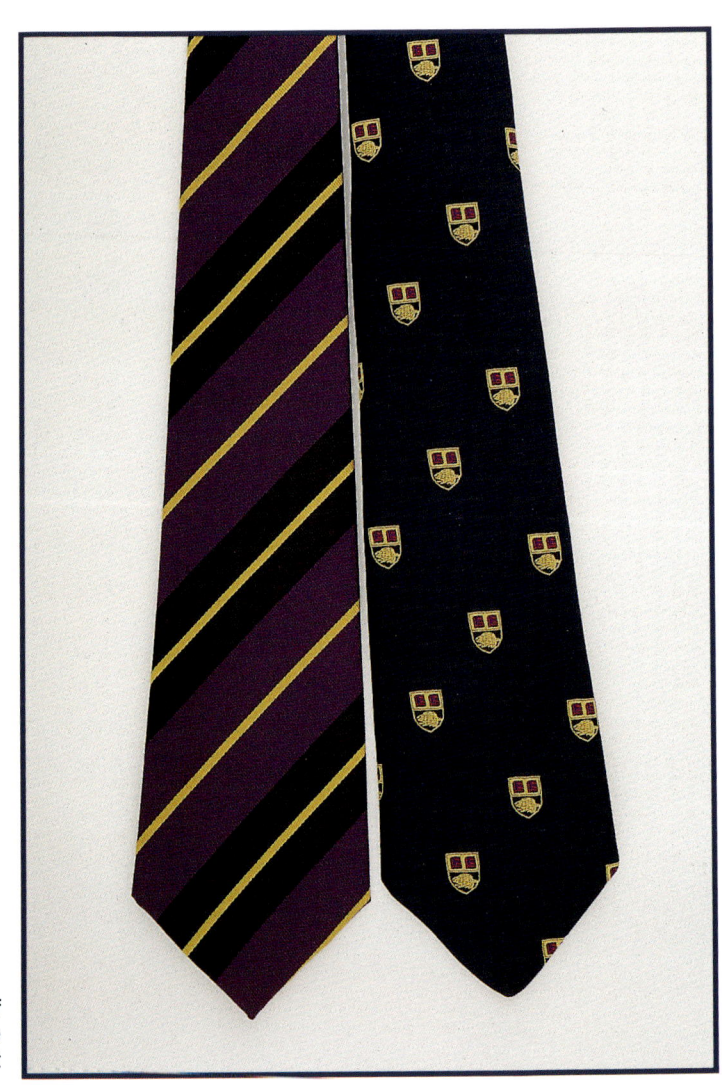

London School of Economics, stripe and crest

80

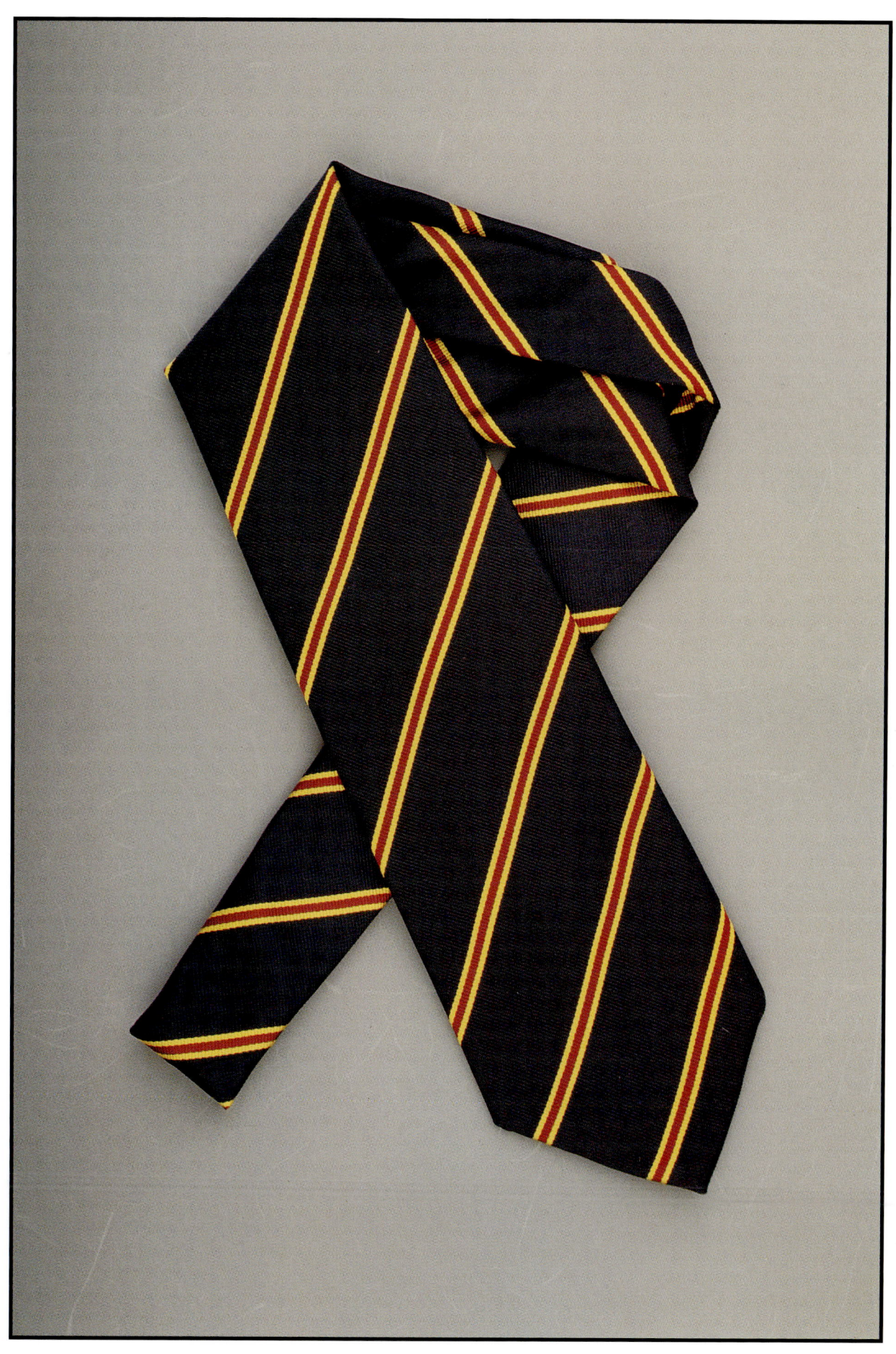

London Hospital

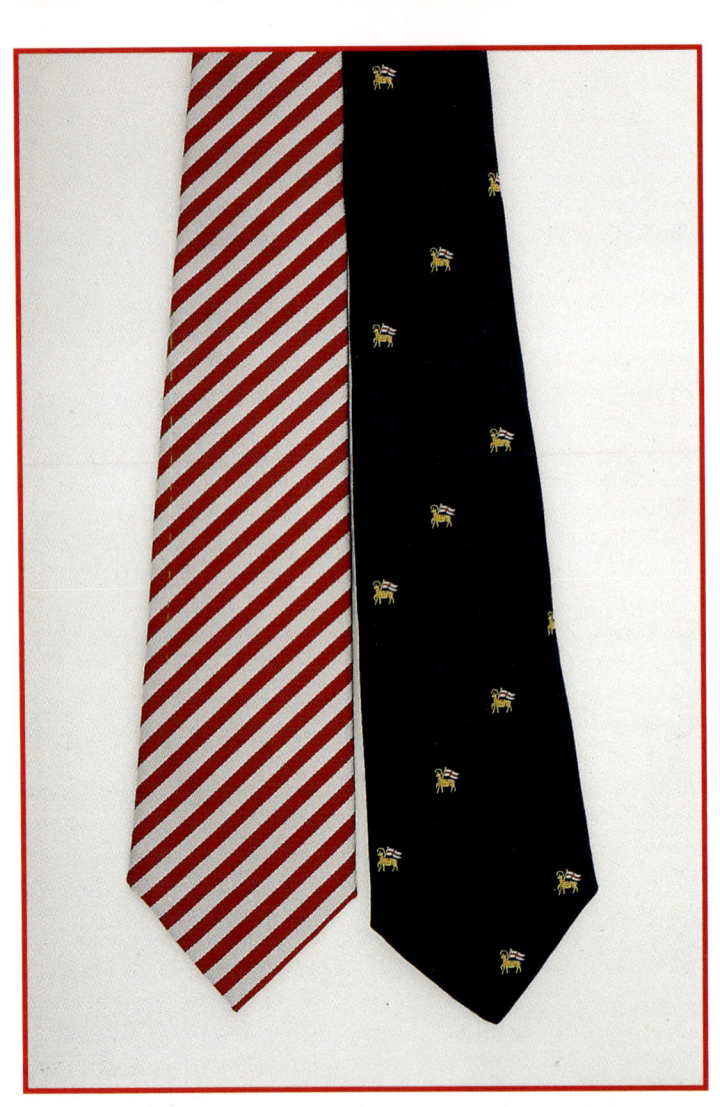

Middle Temple, stripe and crest

St. Bartholomew's Hospital;
St. Thomas's Hospital;
University College

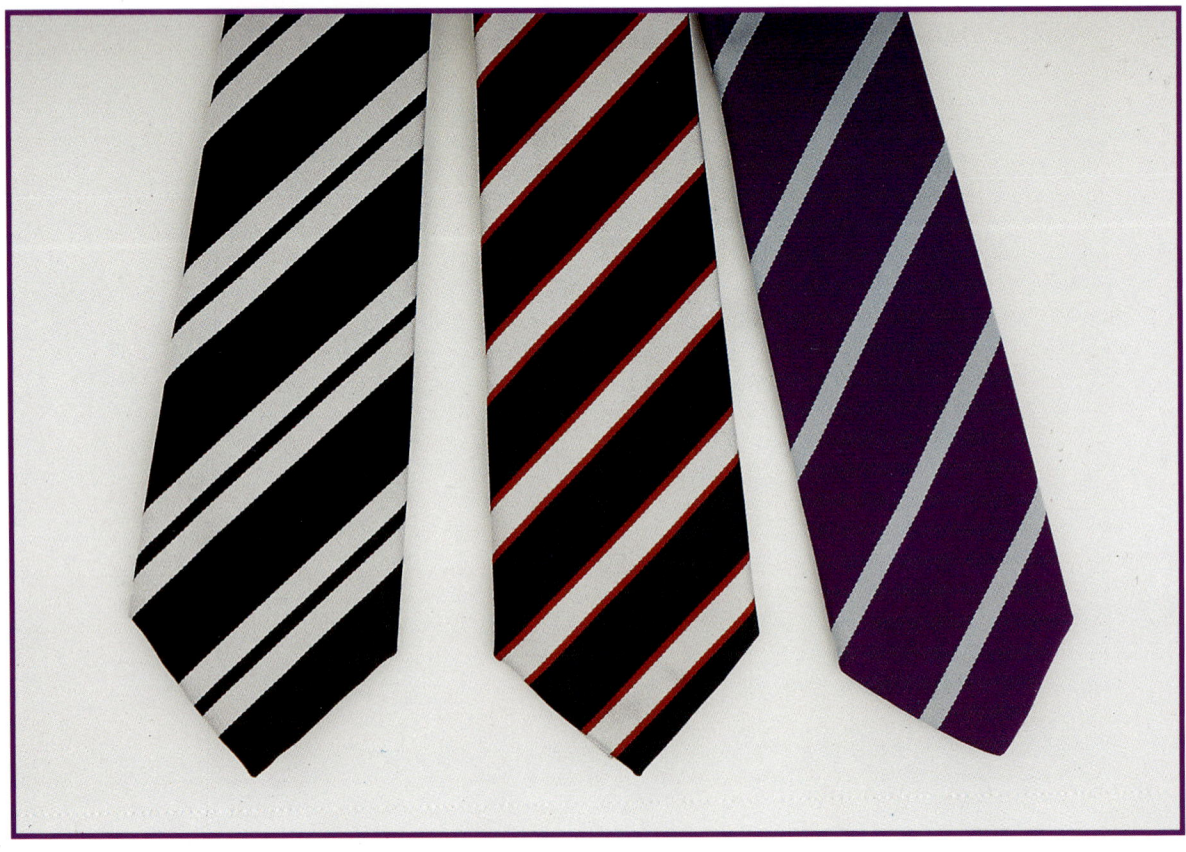

82

Oxford Colleges

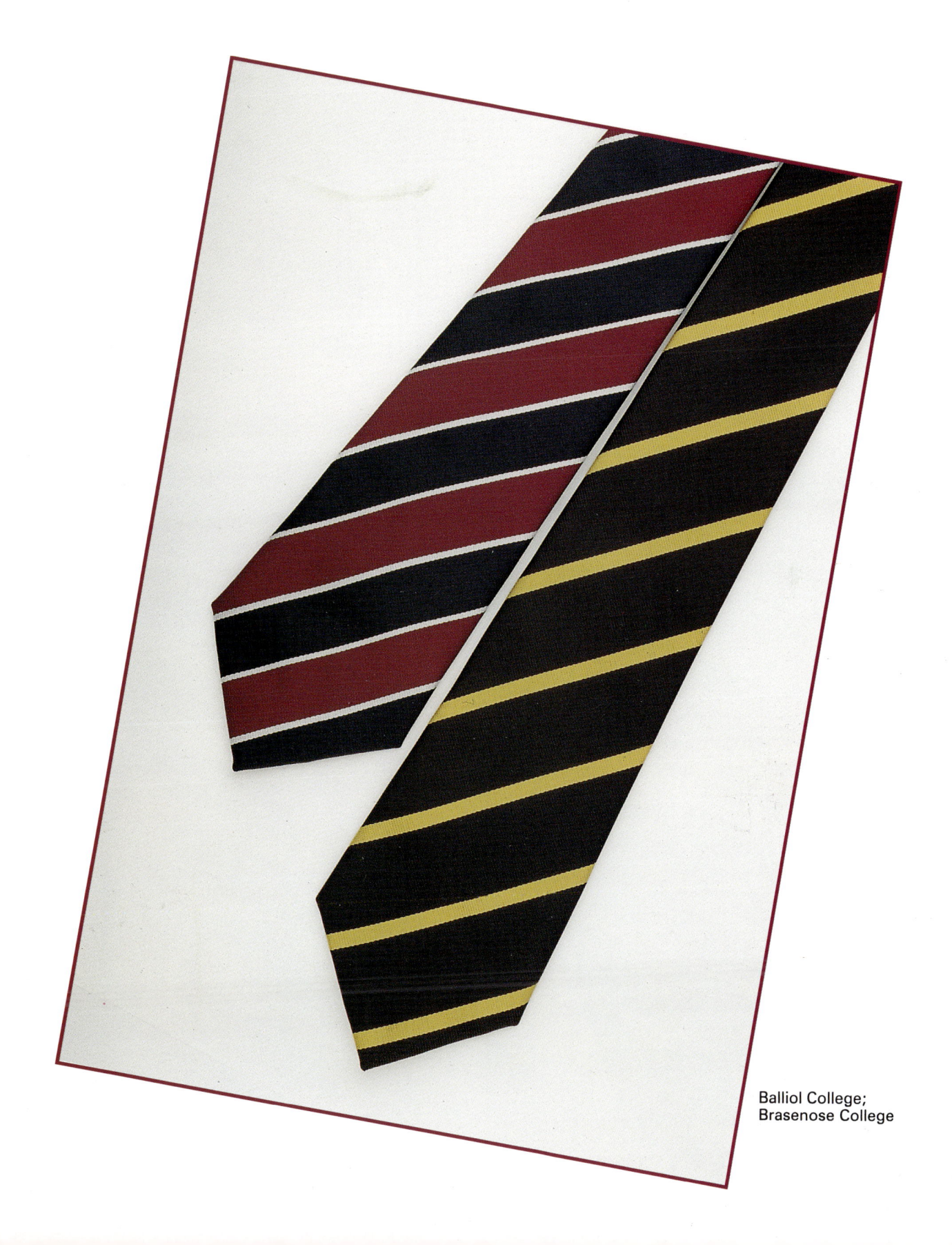

Balliol College;
Brasenose College

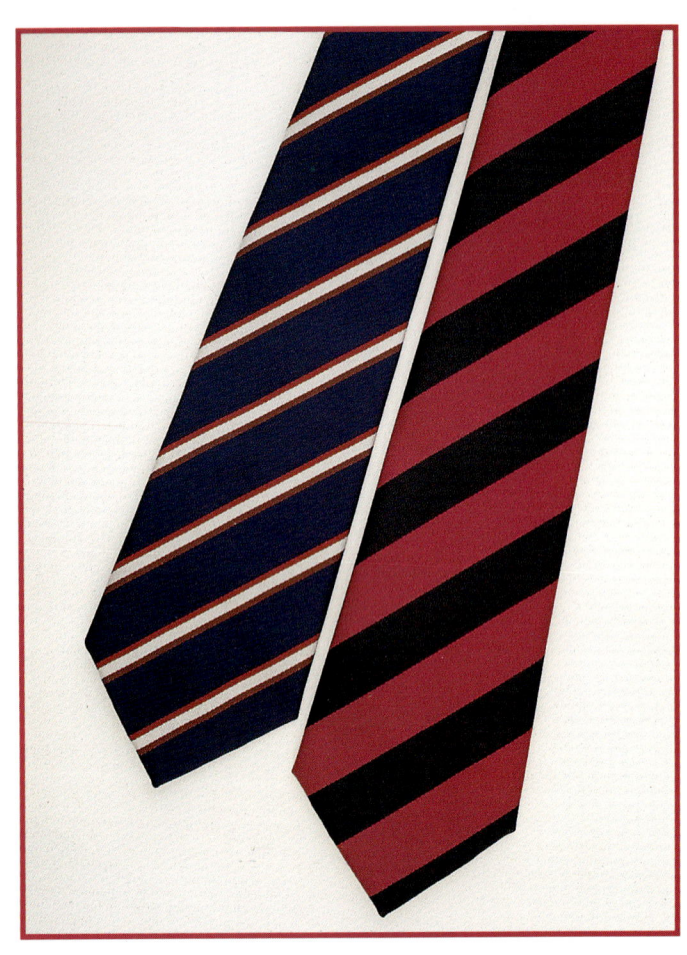

Christ Church College; Corpus Christi College

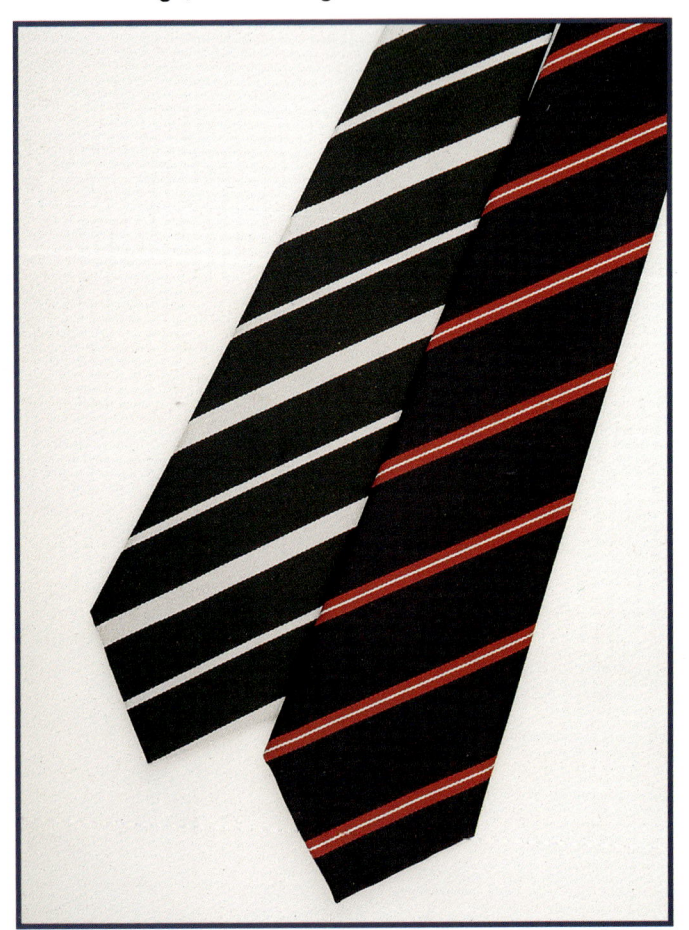

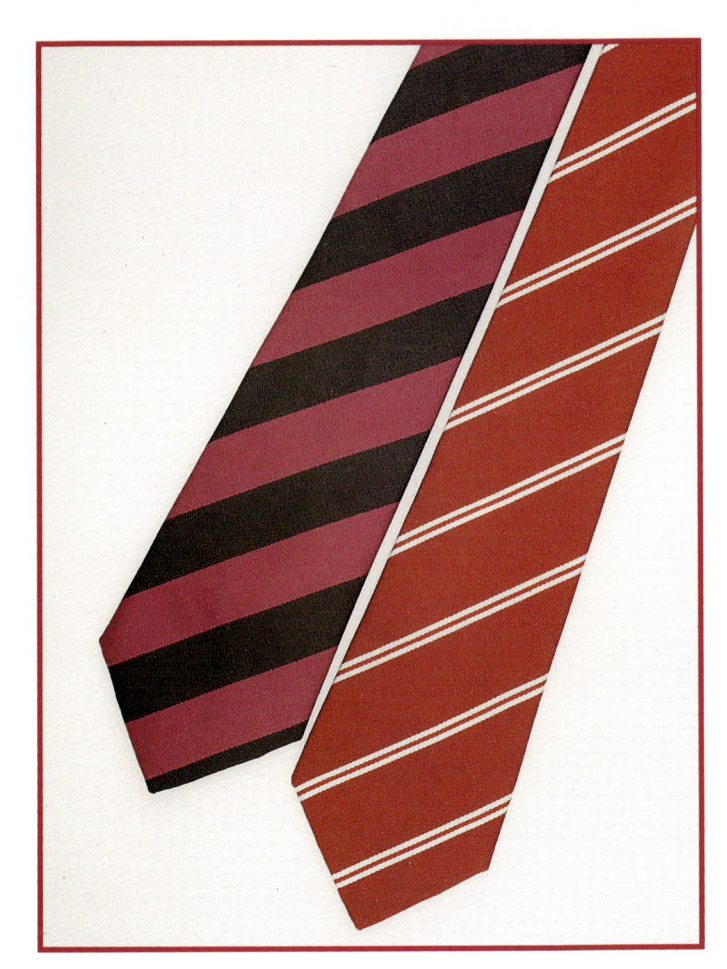

Exeter College; Hertford College

Jesus College; Keble College

Lady Margaret Hall; Lincoln College

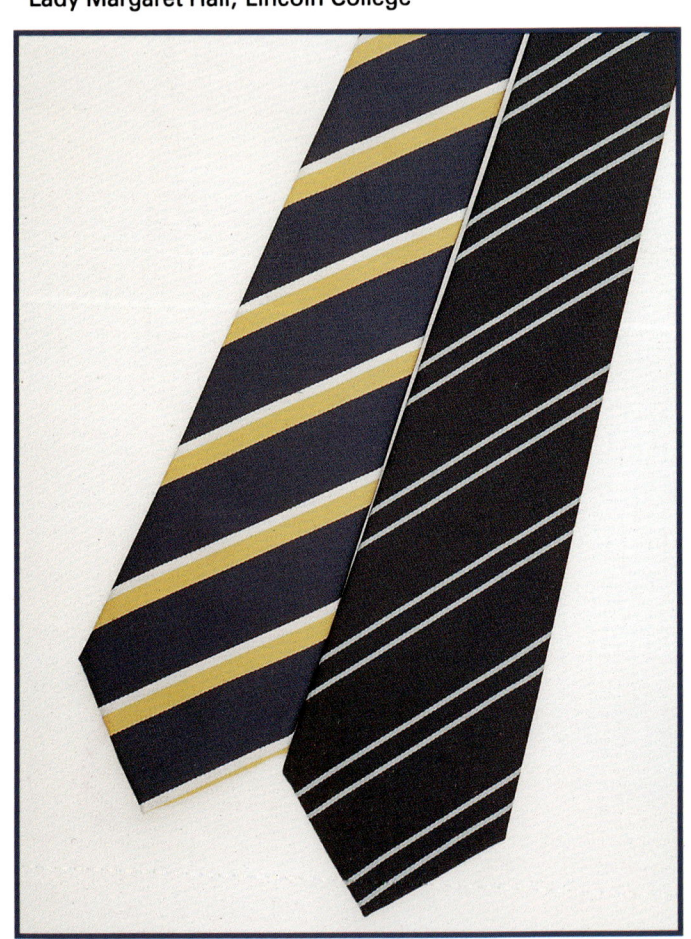

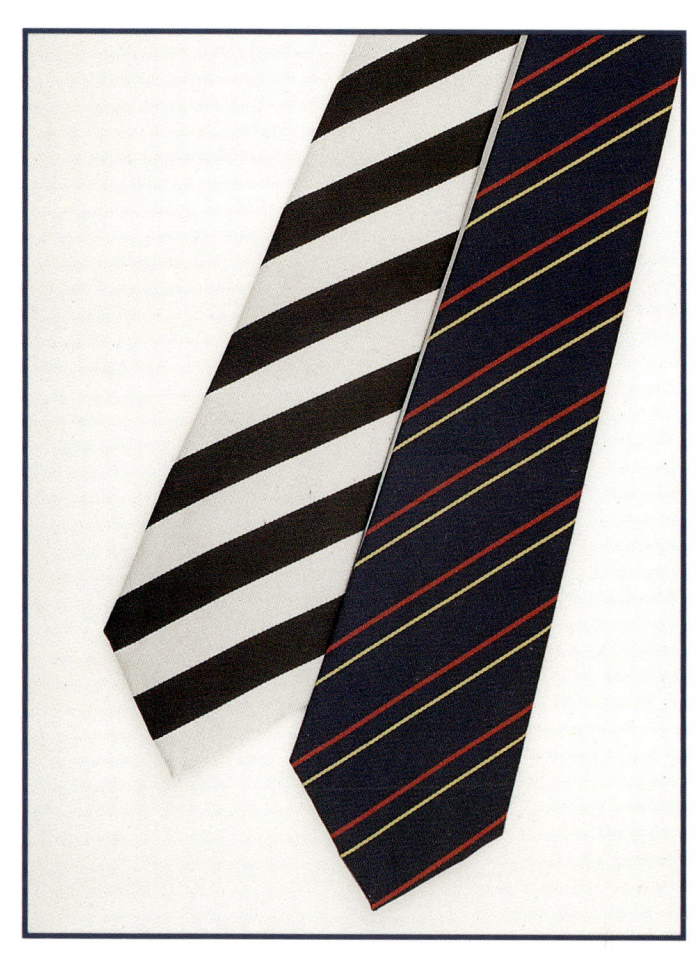

Magdalen College; Mansfield College

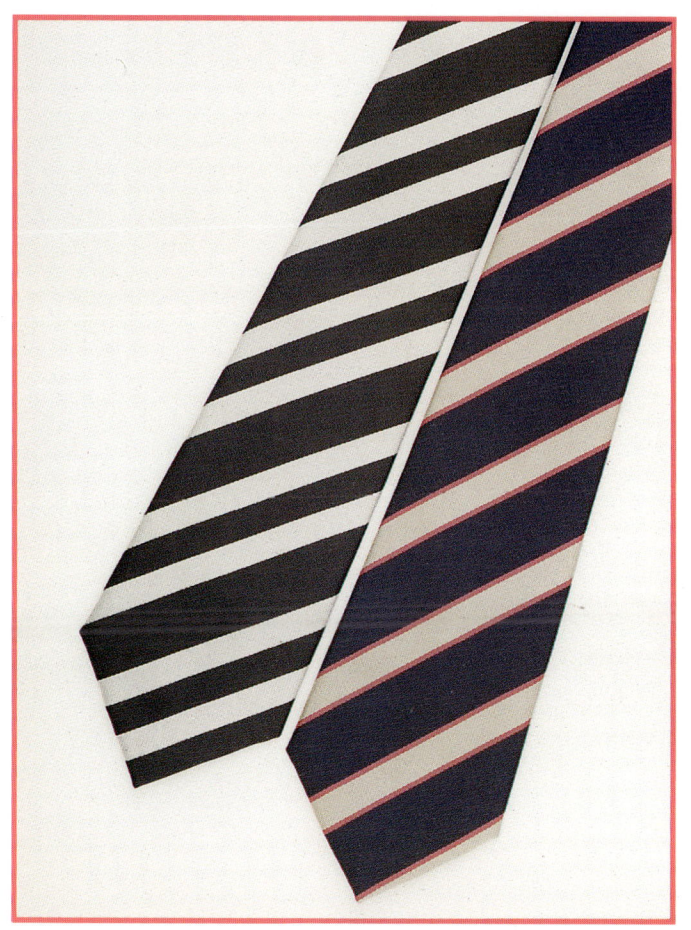

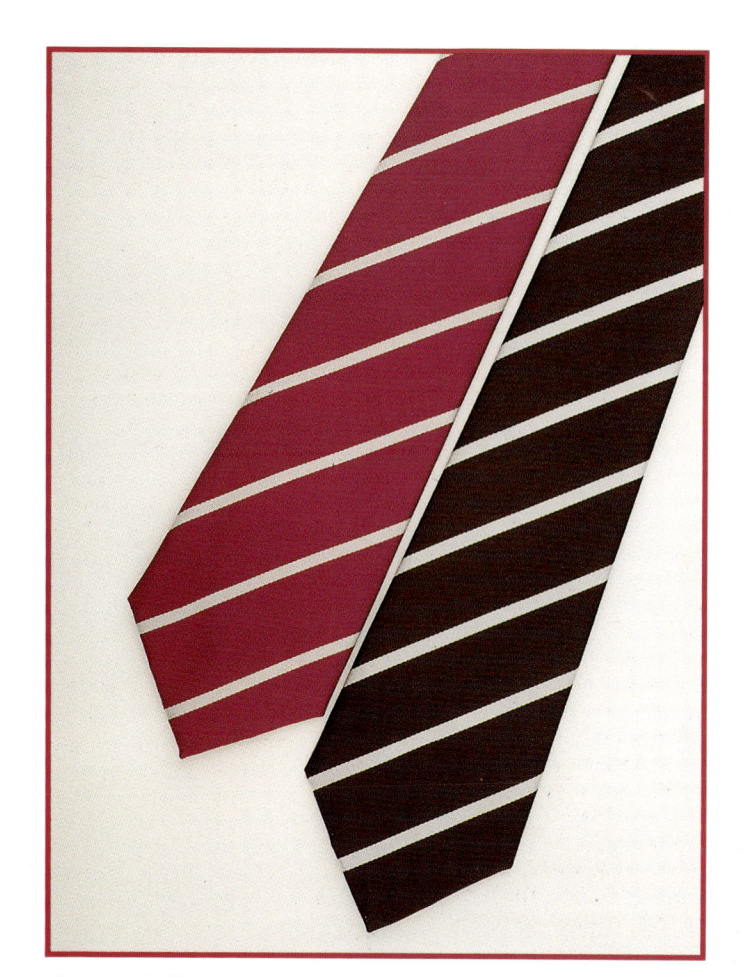

Merton College; New College

Oriel College; Pembroke College

Queen's College; St. Anne's College

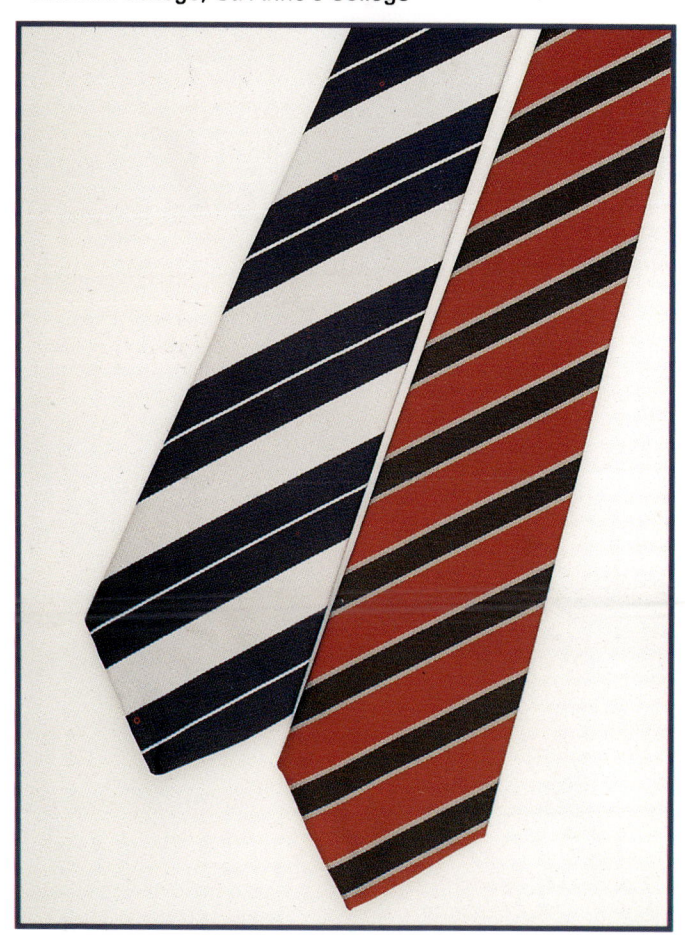

85

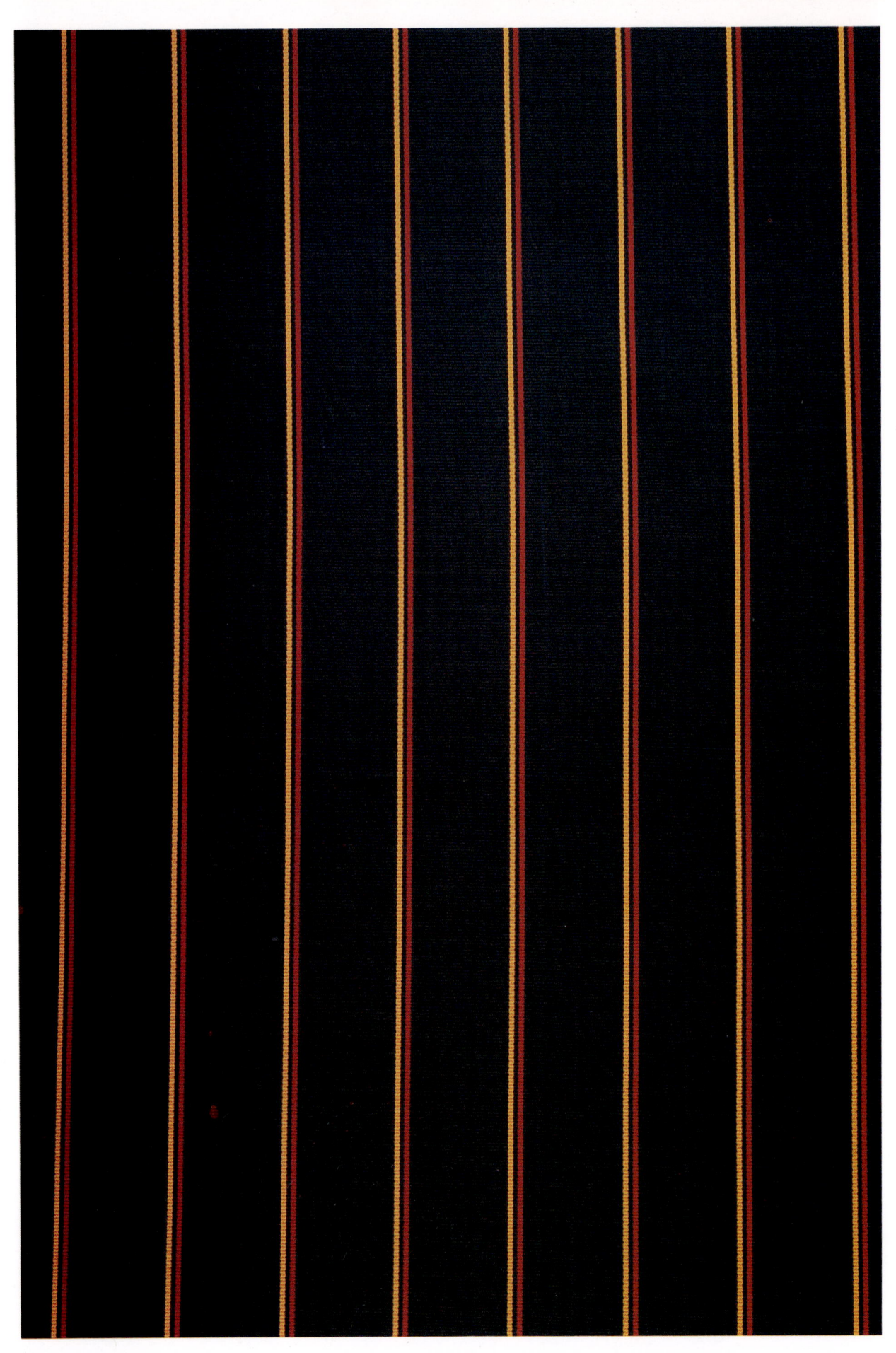

St. Anthony's College, swatch

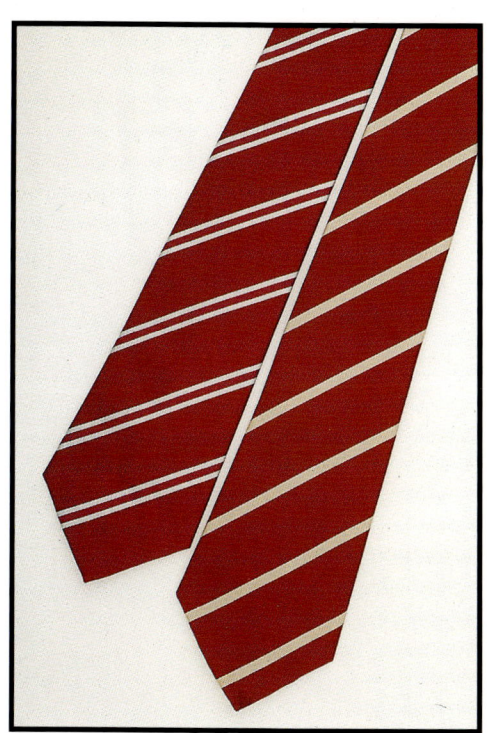

St. Catherine's College; St. Edmund Hall

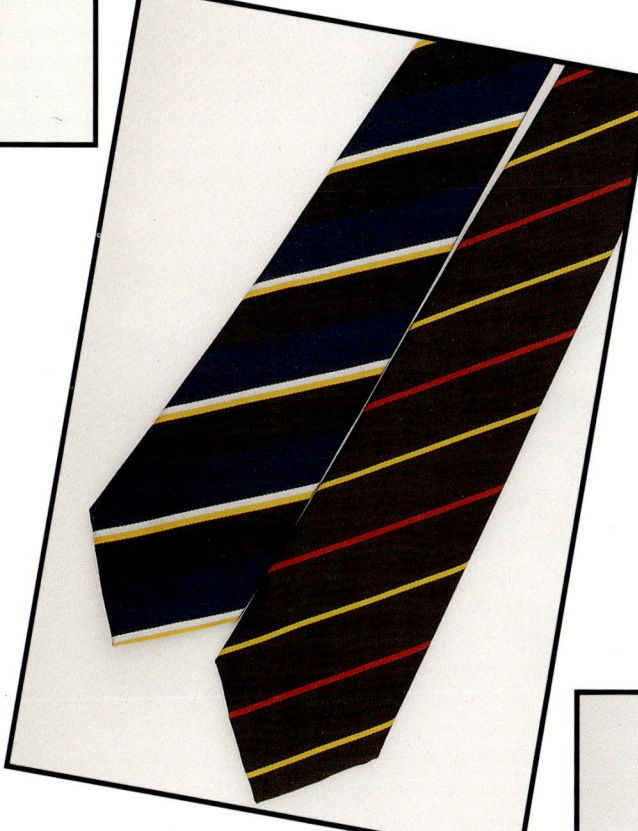

St. Hugh's College; St. John's College

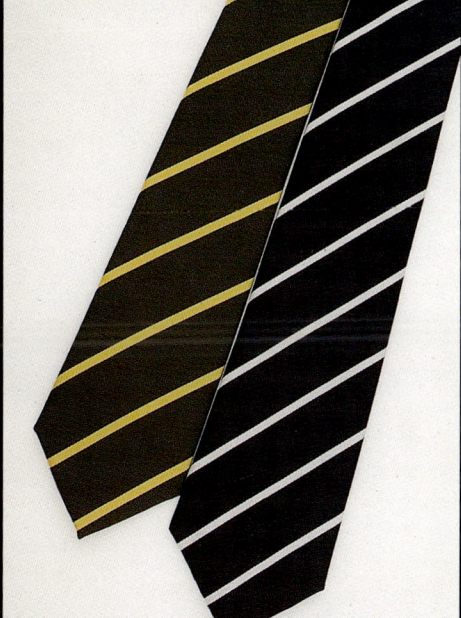

St. Peter's College; Trinity College

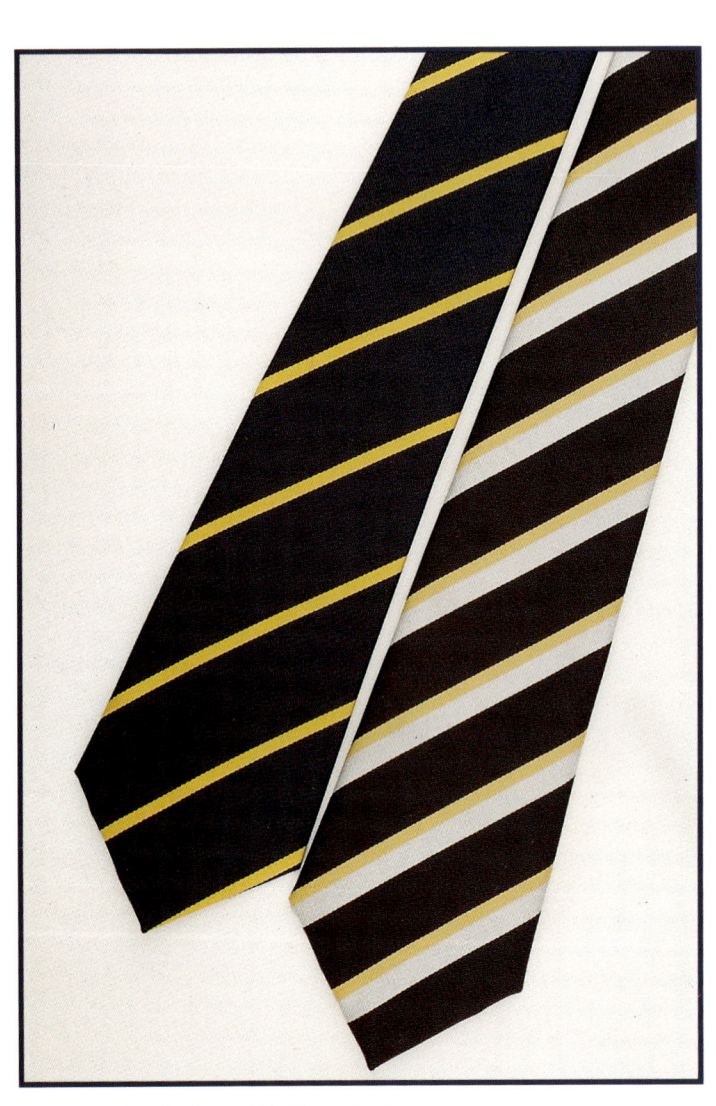

University College; Wadham College

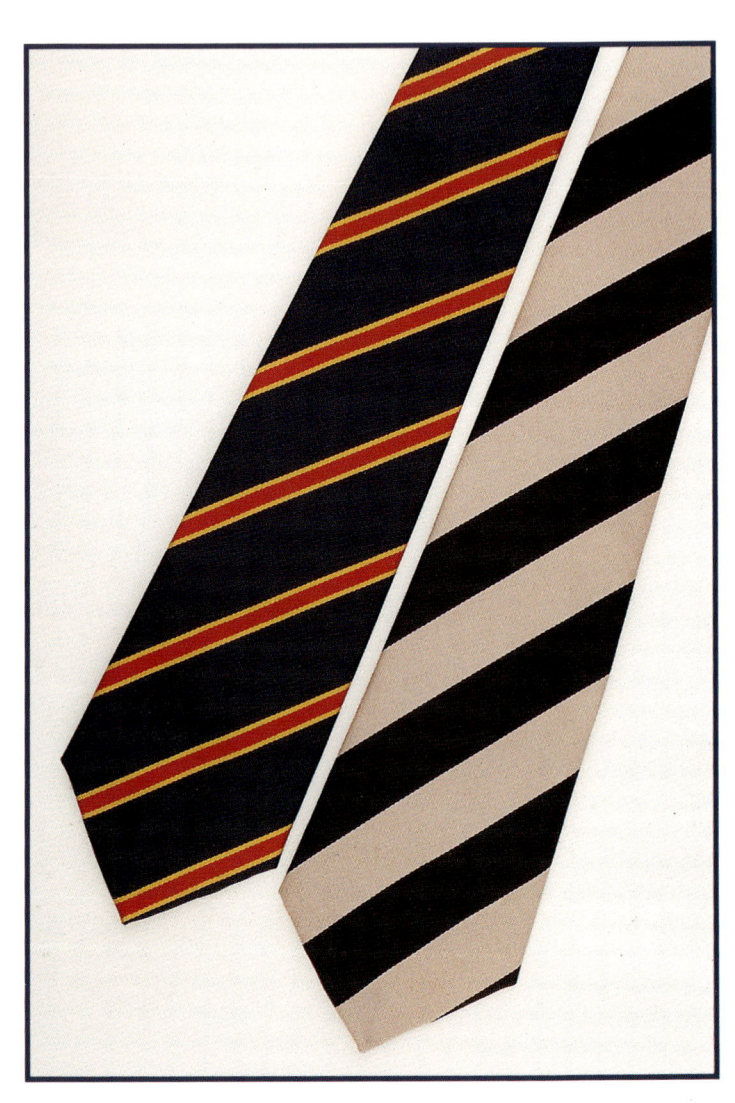

Wolfson College; Worcester College

Old Boys

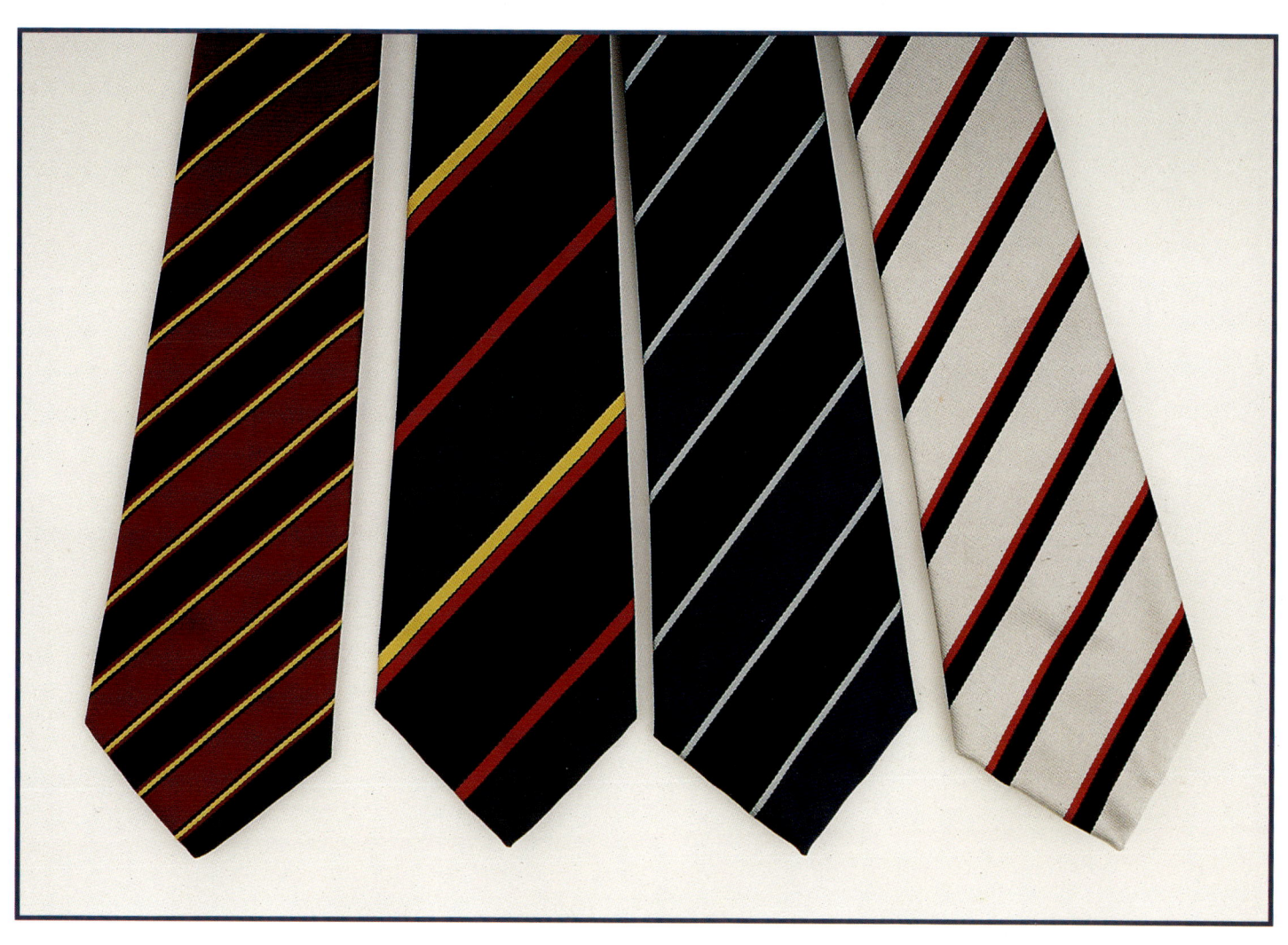

Old Albanian; Old Aldenham; Old Alleynian (Dulwich College); Old Ampleforth

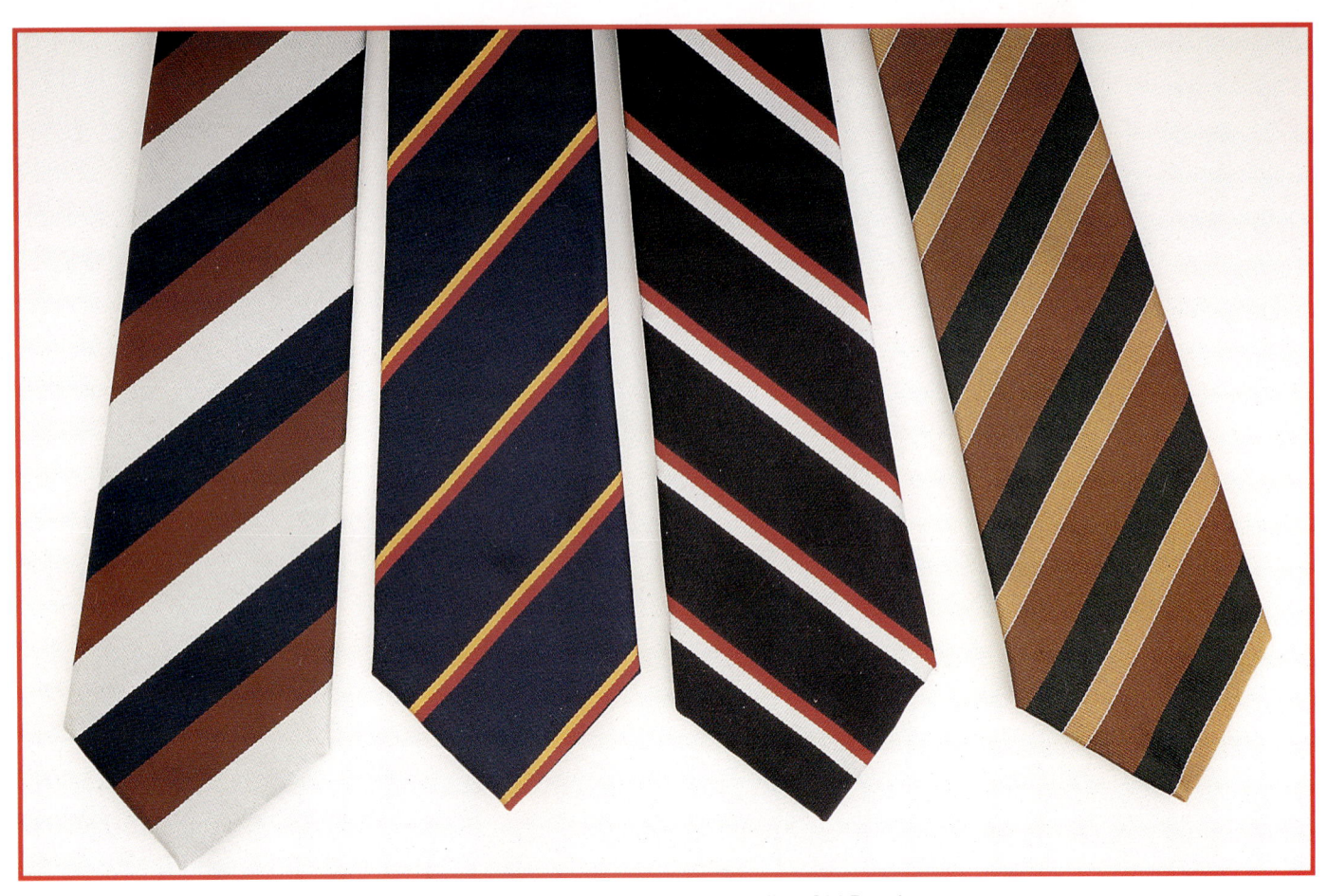

Old Beaumont; Old Blues; Old Blundell's; Old Bootham
Old Bradfield; Old Brentwood; Old Bristol; Old Canford

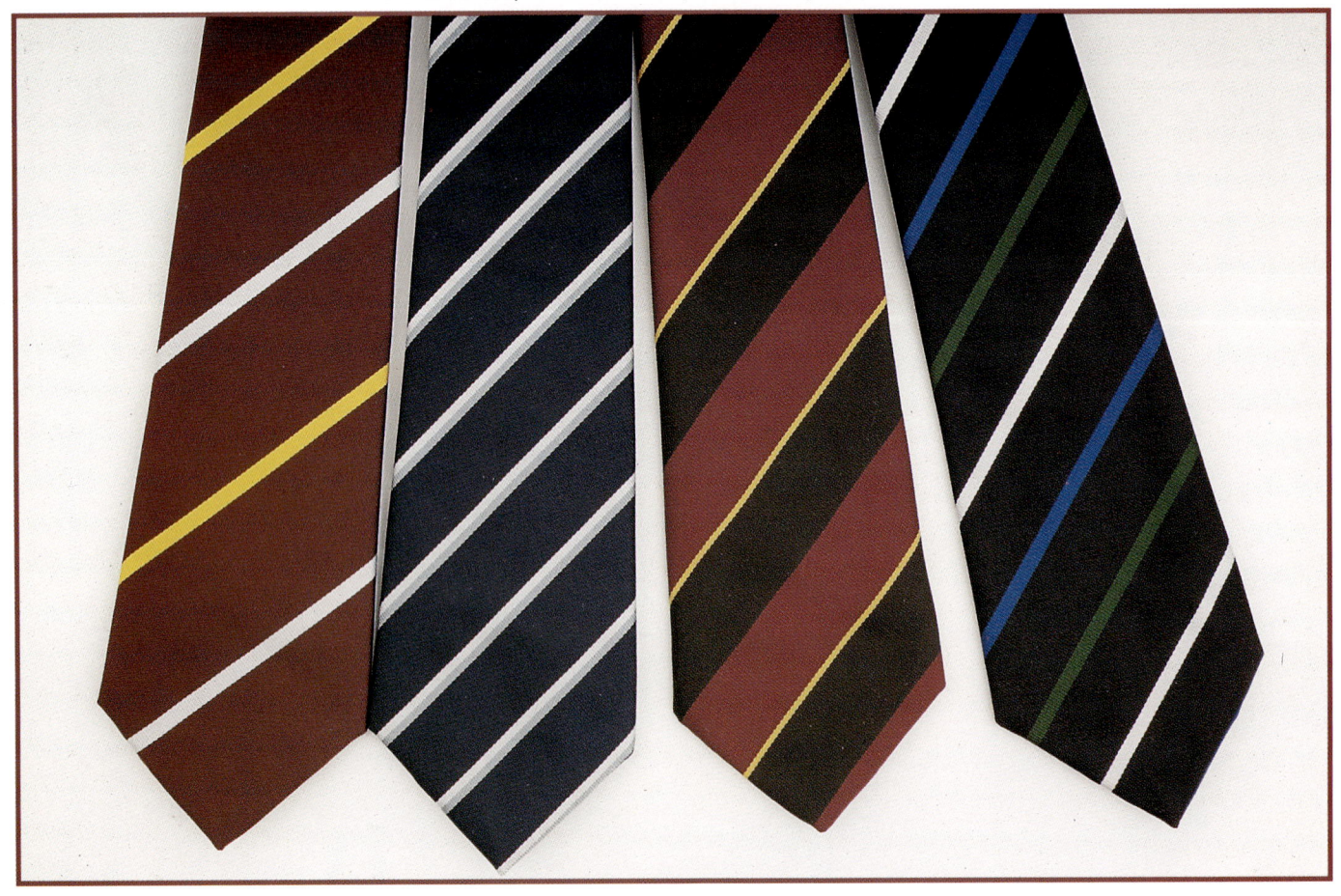

90

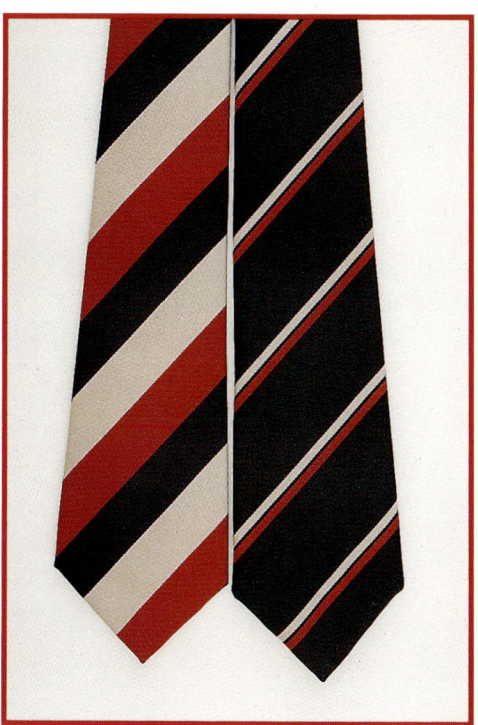

Old Carthusian, wide and narrow stripes

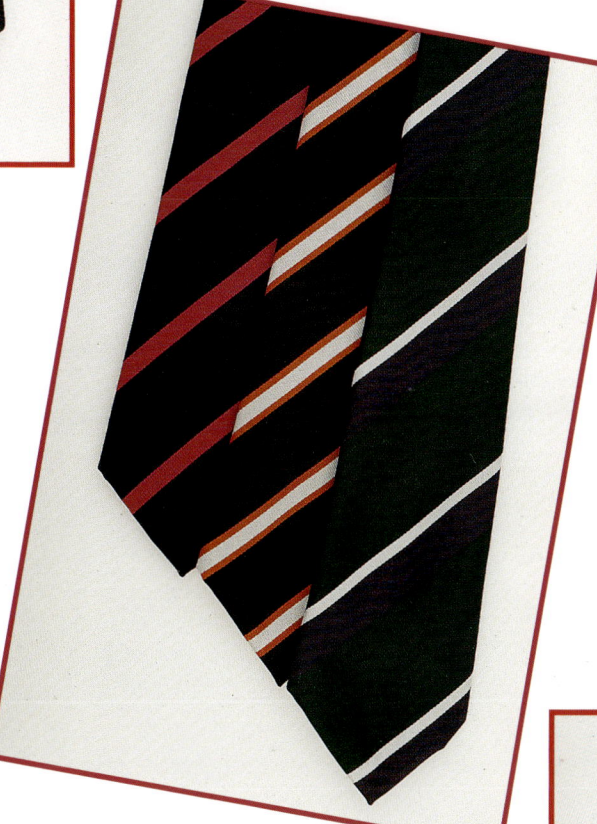

Old Cheltonian; Old Citizens (City of London); Old Clifton

Old Dovorian, wide and narrow stripes

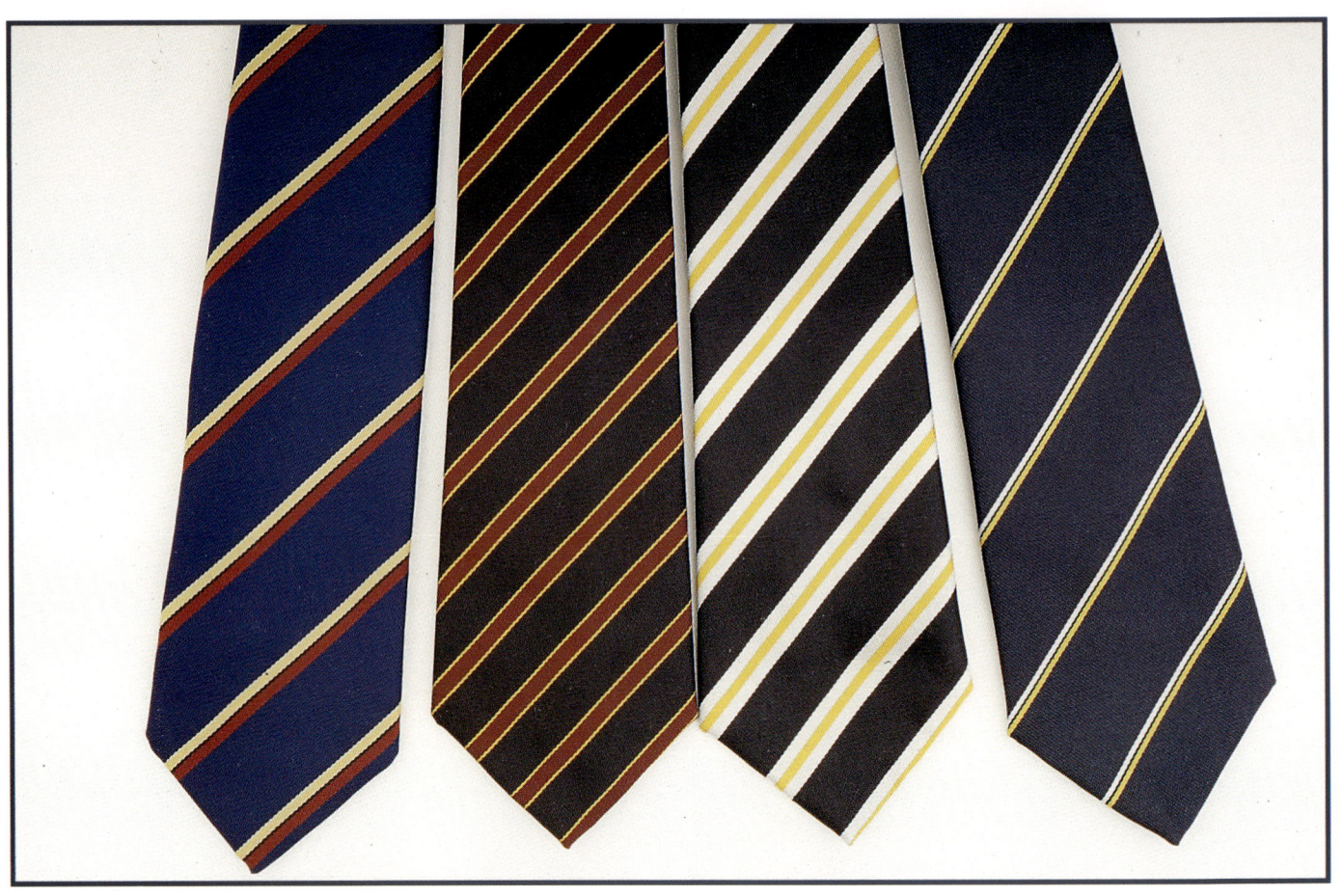

Old Edwardian (New Street Birmingham); Old Downside; Old Elean (King's School, Ely); Old Emanuel (Wandsworth)

Old Epsom; Old Eton; Old Felsted; Old Glenalmond

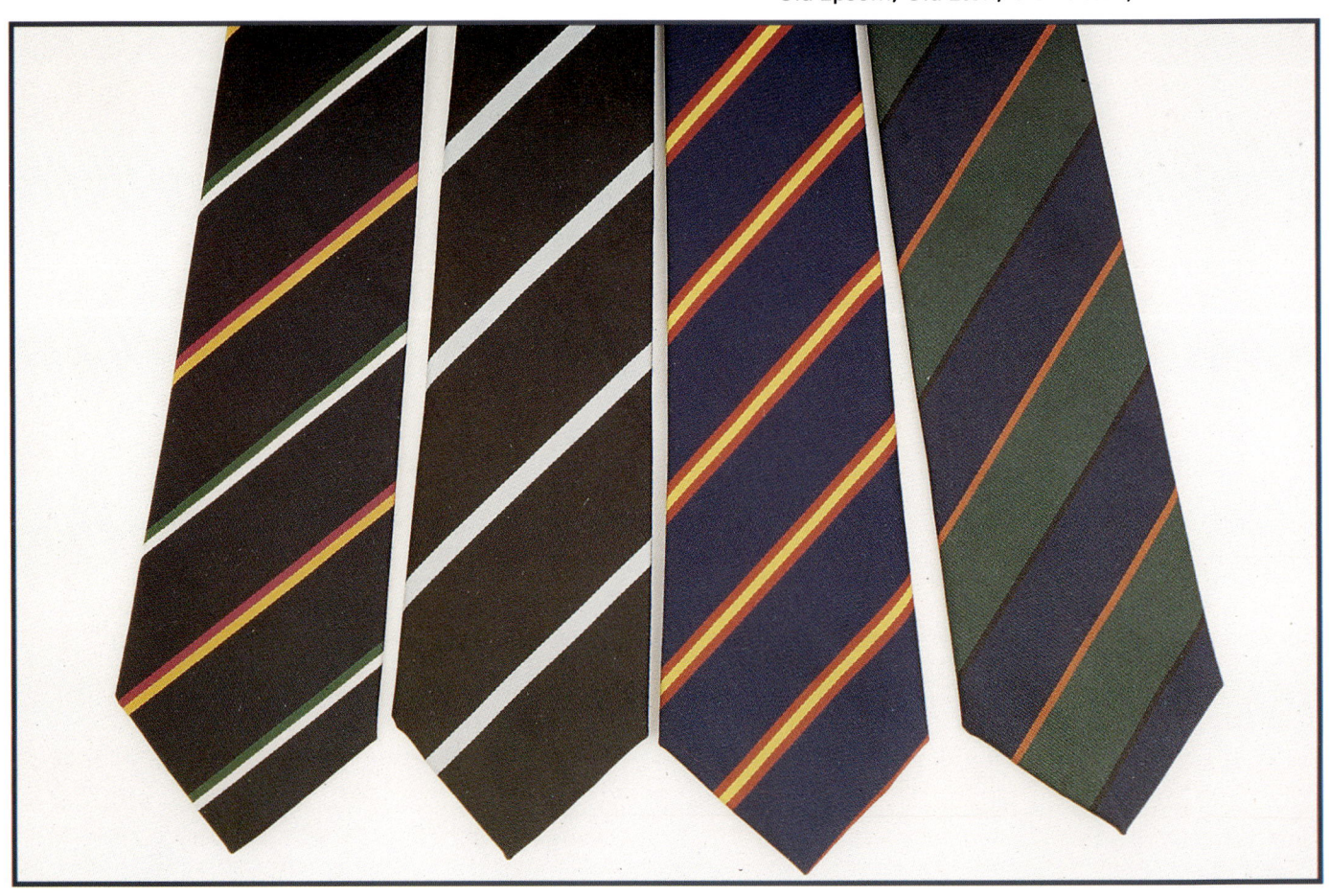

92

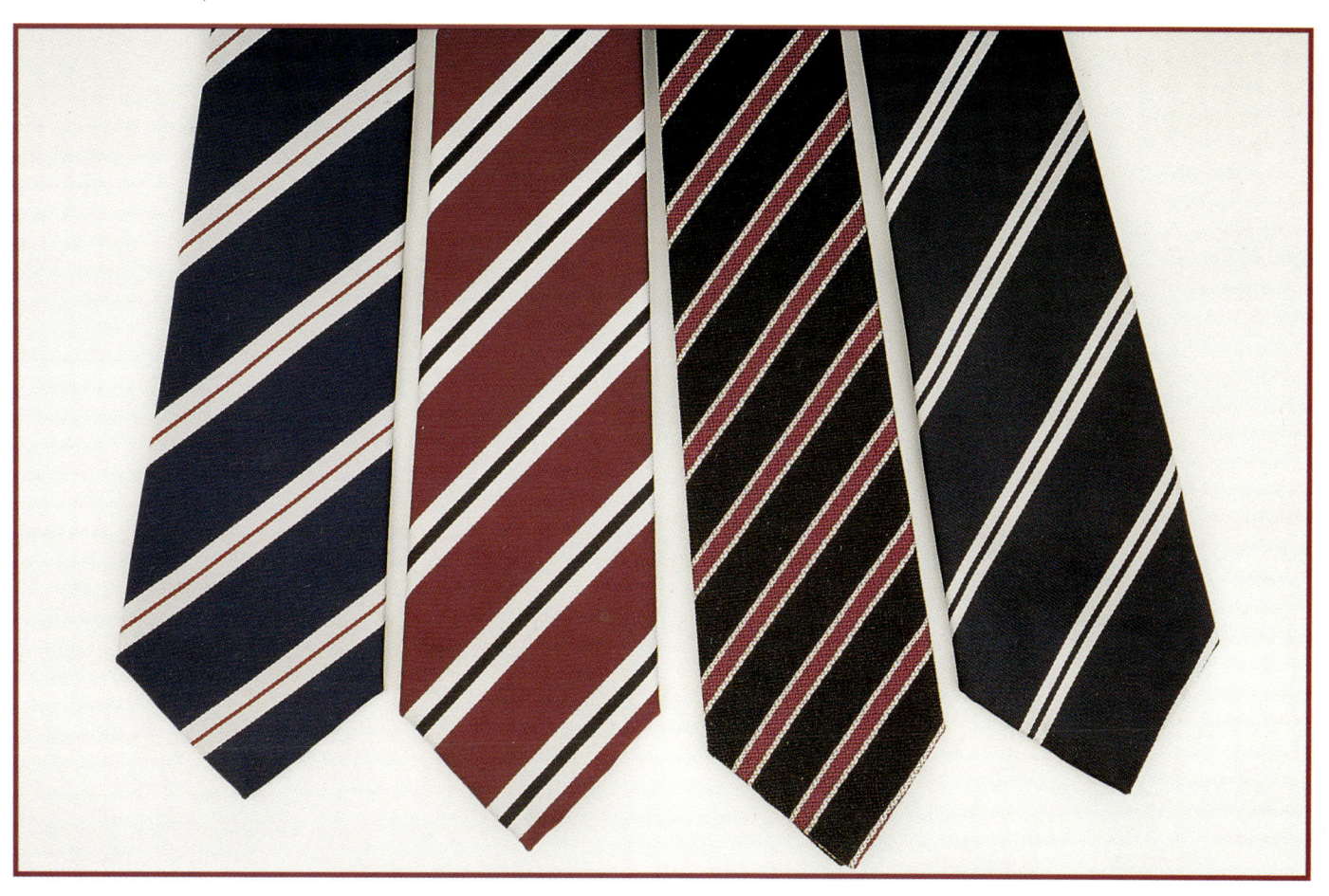

Old Haberdashers; Old Haileybury, majenta; Old Haileybury, black; Old Harrow

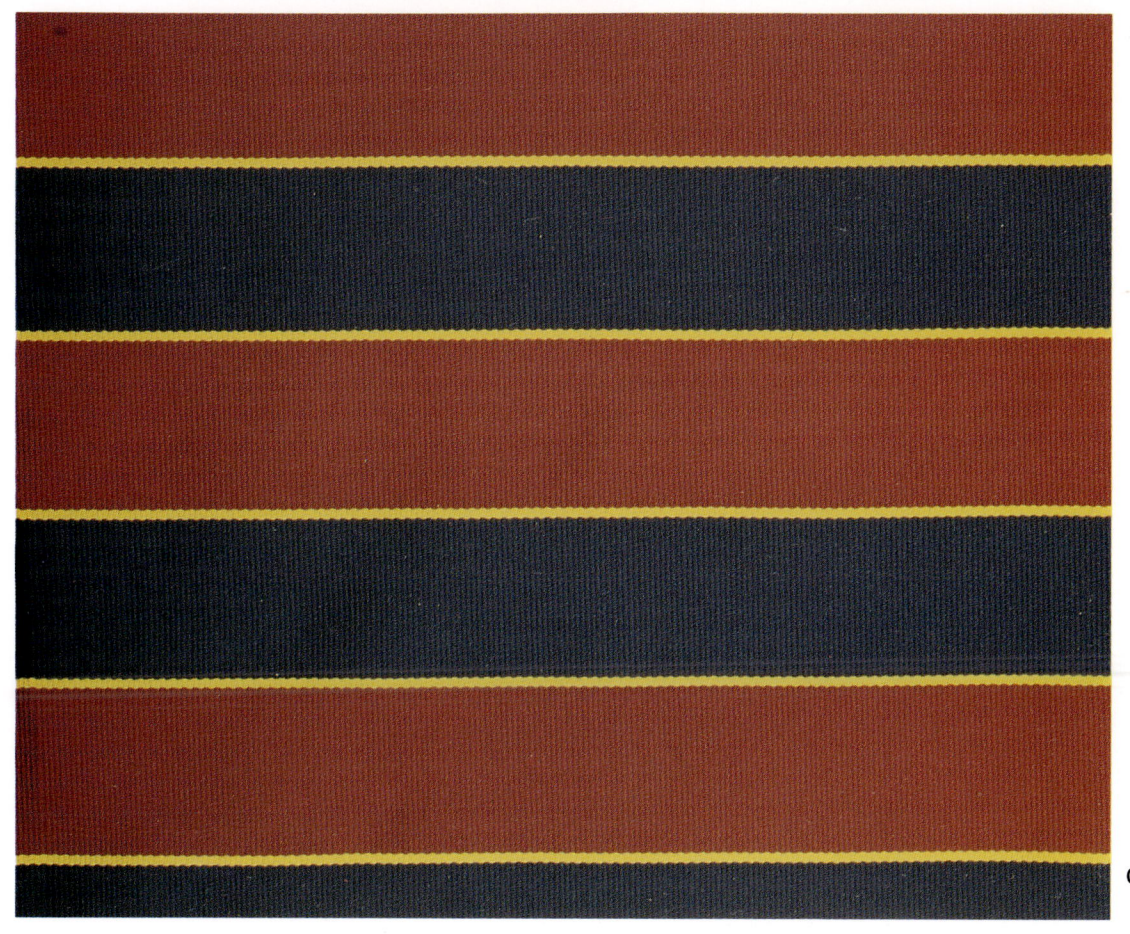

Old Helean, swatch

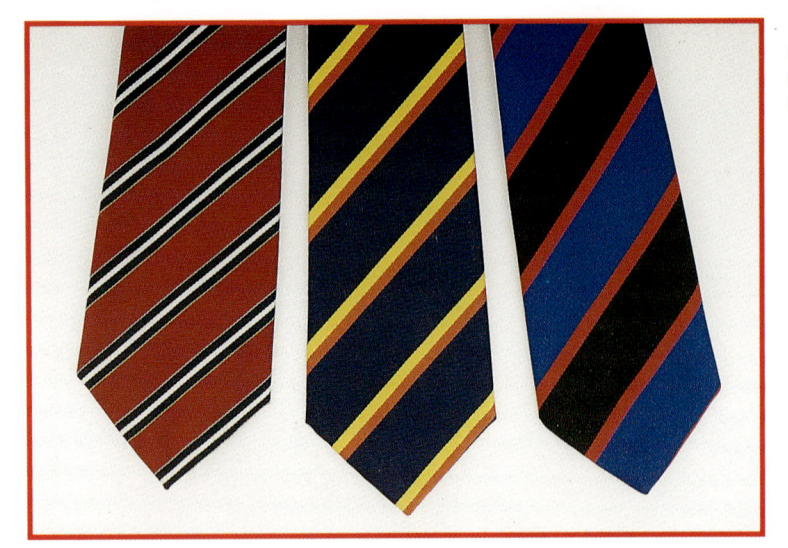

Old King's Canterbury;
Old King's Wimbledon;
Old Lancastrian

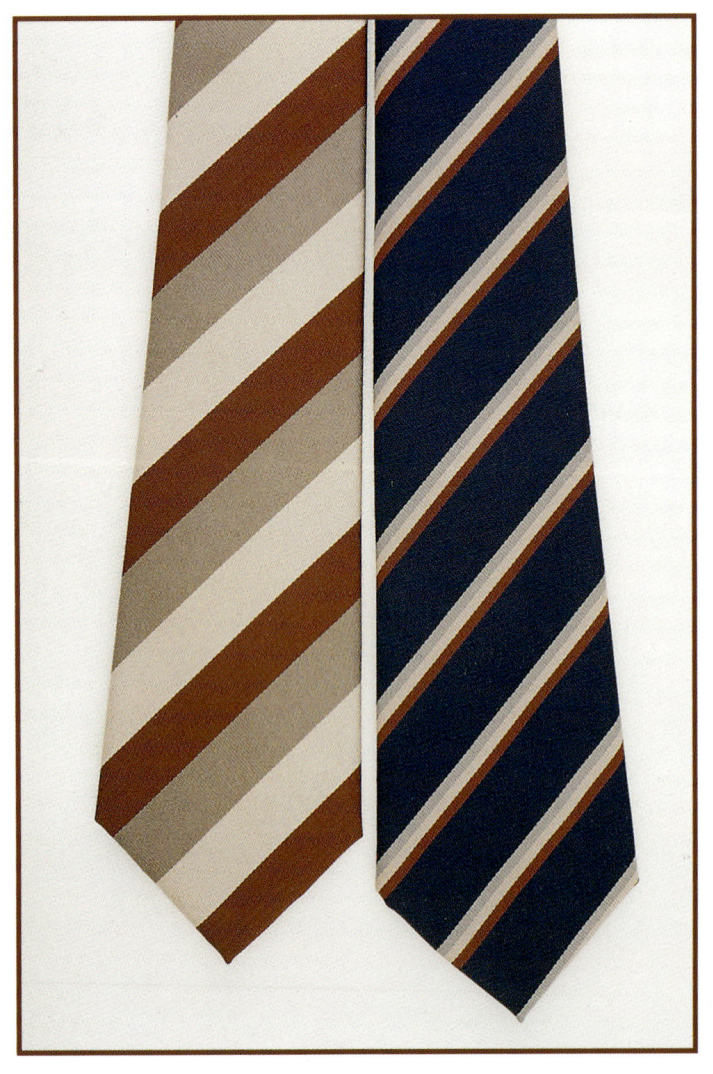

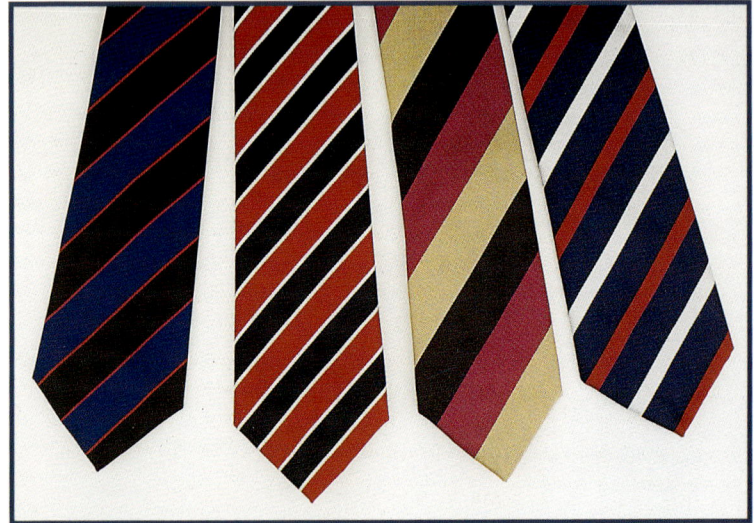

Old Malvern; Old Marlborough; Old Merchant Taylors'; Old Oundle

Old Lancing, wide and narrow stripes

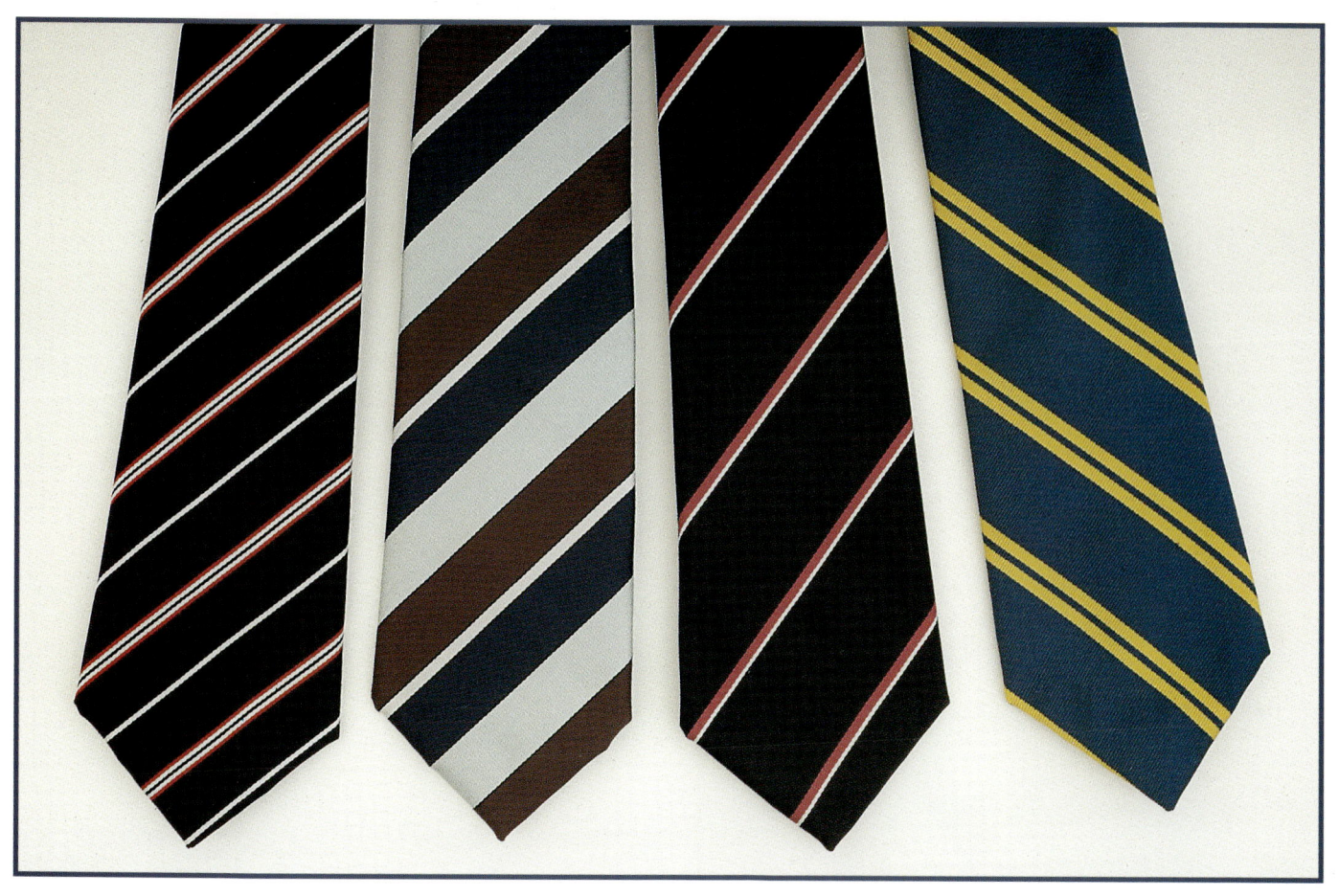

Old Pauline; Old Peterite; Old Radley; Old Repton

Old Rossall; Old Rugby

Old Salopian, wide and narrow stripes

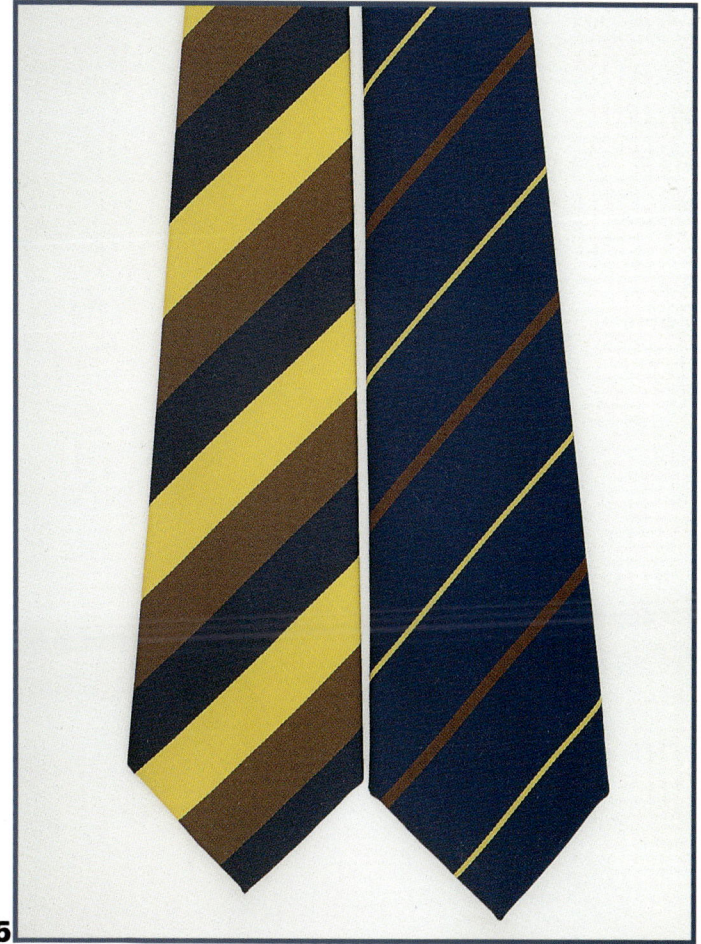

95

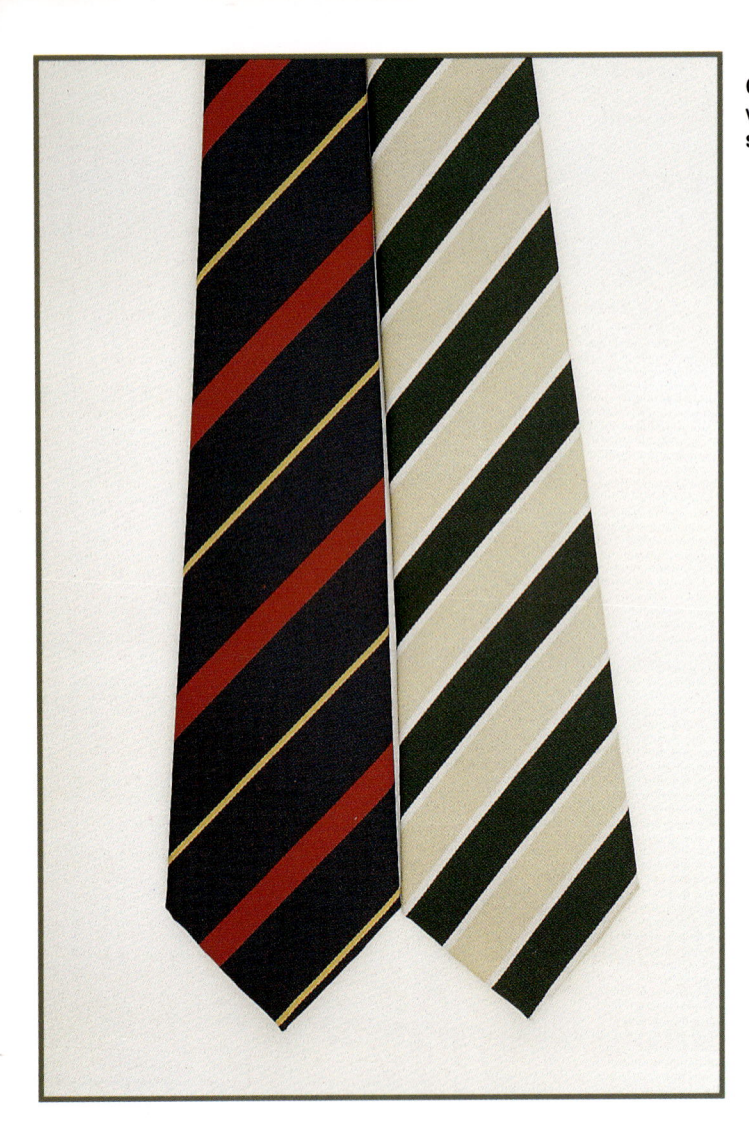

Old Sherborne,
wide and narrow
stripes

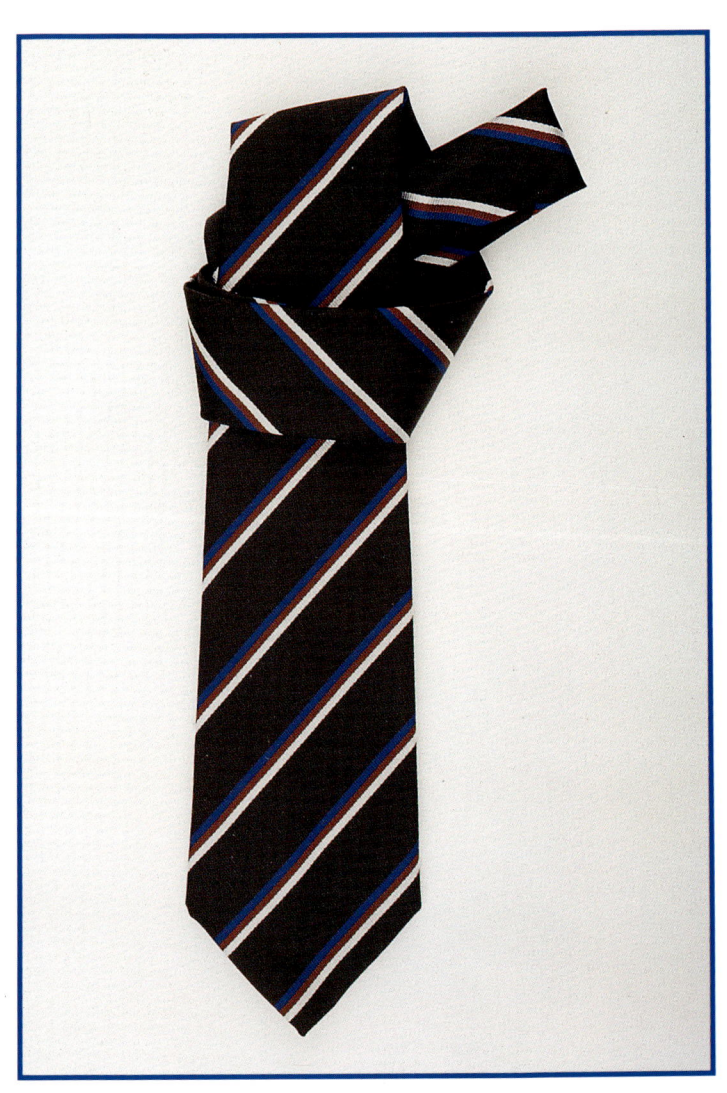

Old Stowe

96

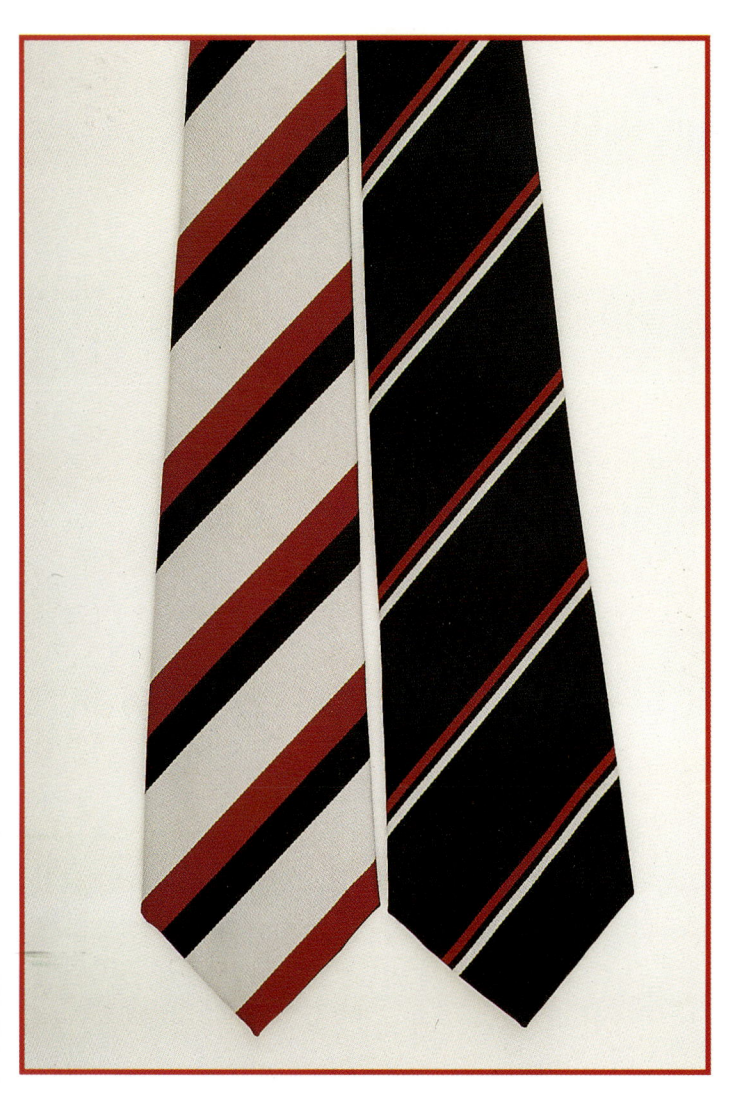

Old Tonbridge, wide and narrow stripes

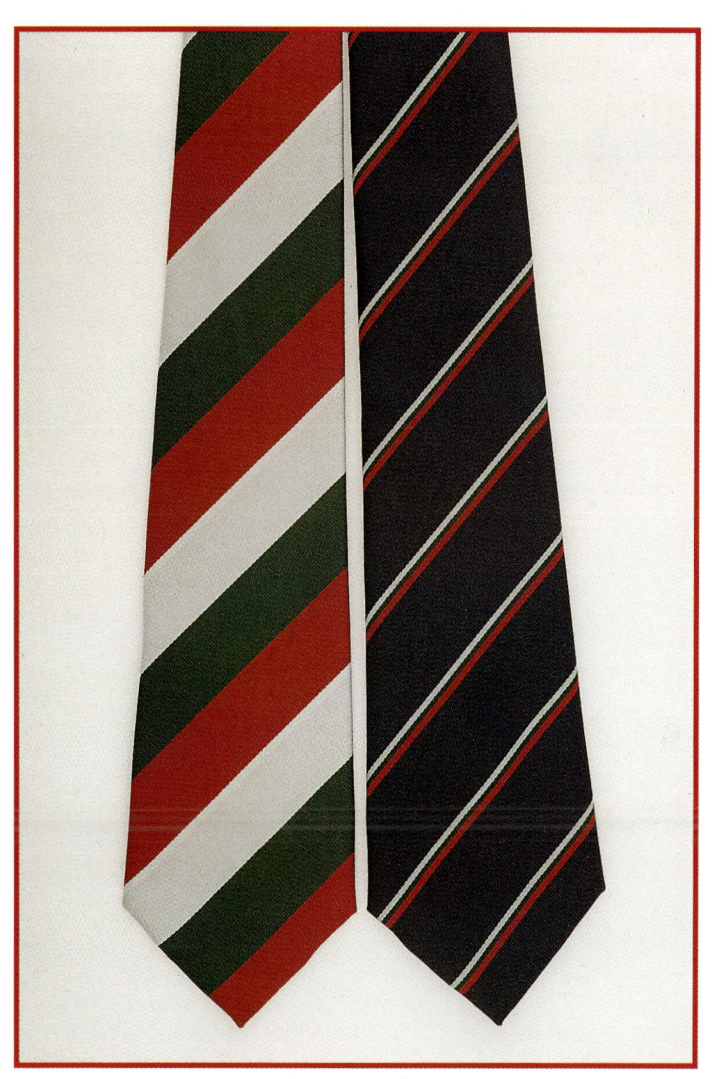

Old Uppingham, wide and narrow stripes

97

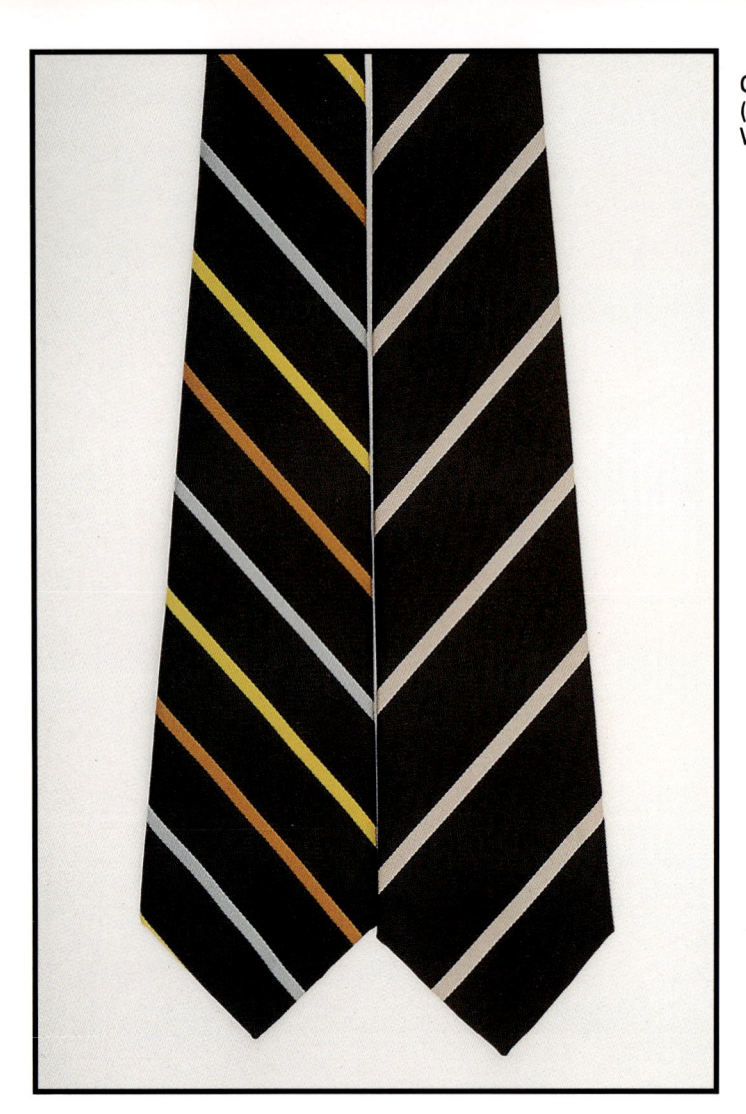

Old Wellington (Berkshire); Old Westminster

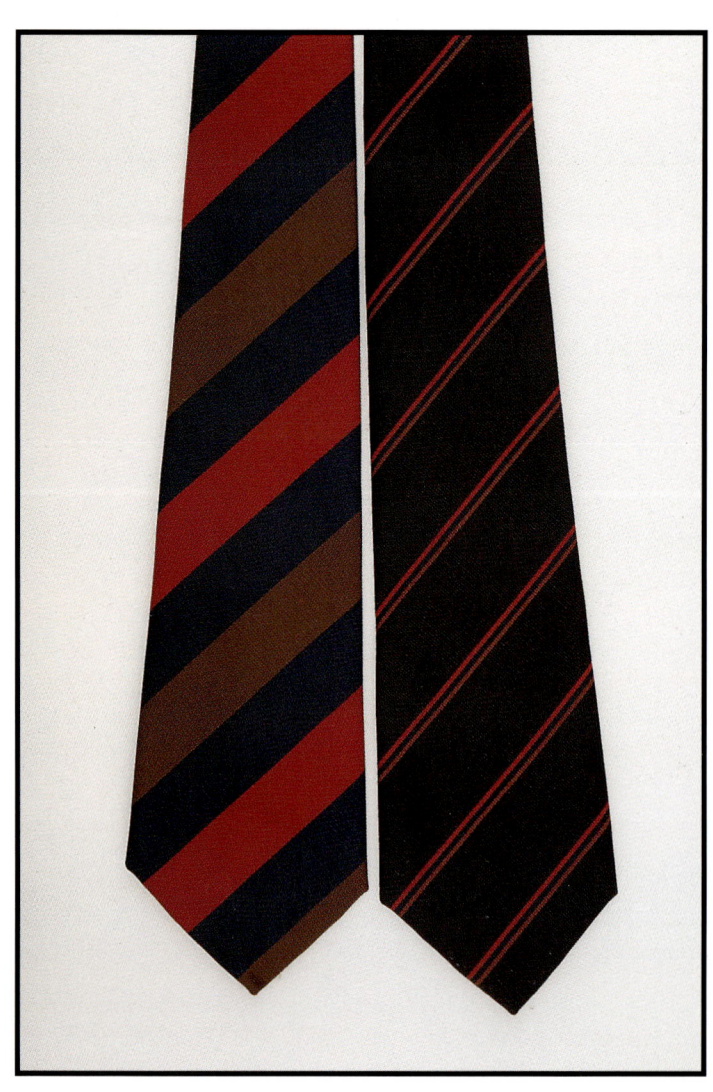

Old Wykehamist, wide and narrow stripes

98

Clubs, etc.

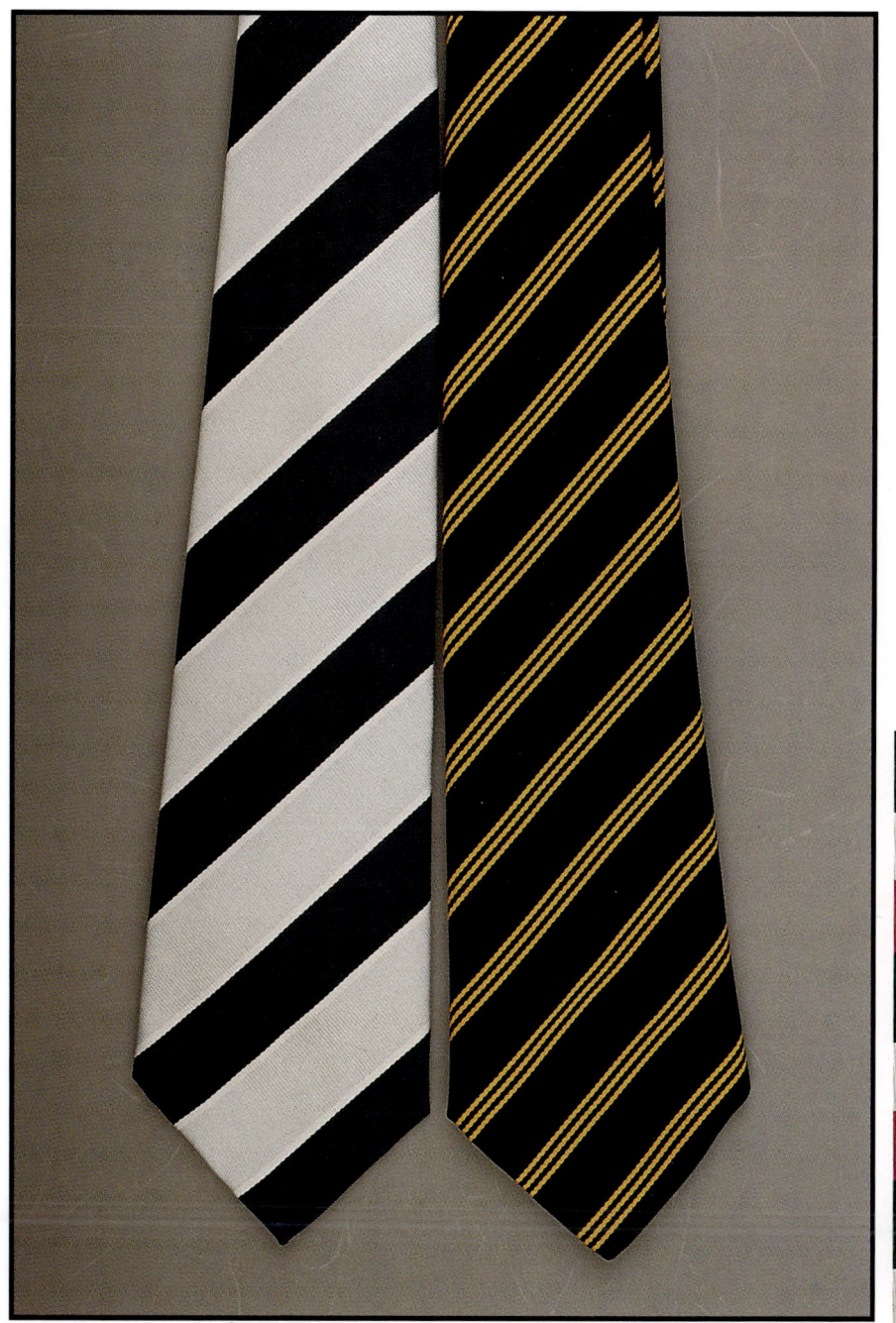

Barbarians R.F.C.;
British Legion

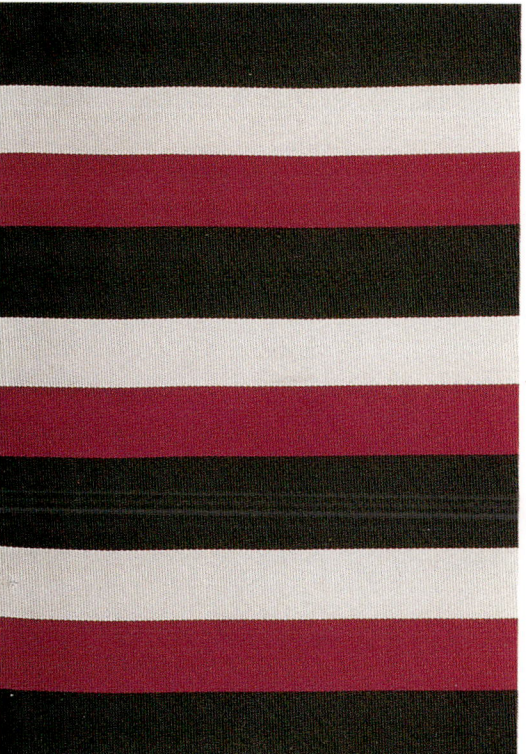

Free Foresters C.C.,
swatch

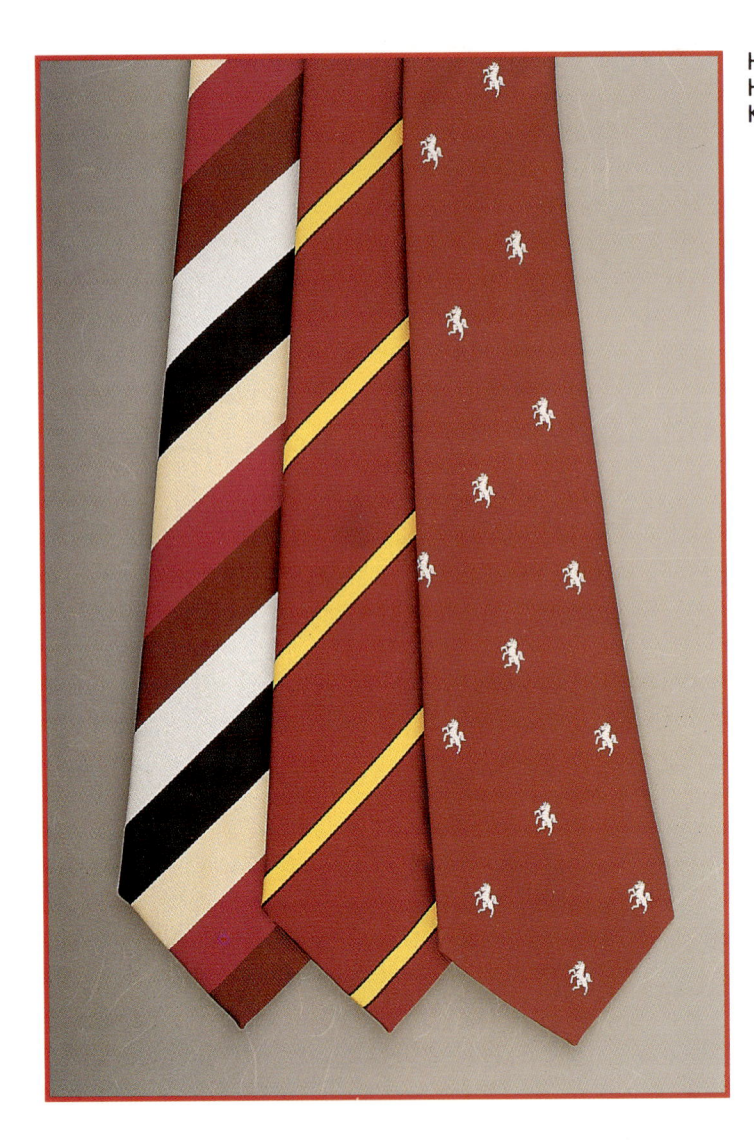

Harlequins R.F.C.;
Hawks, Cambridge;
Kent County C.C.

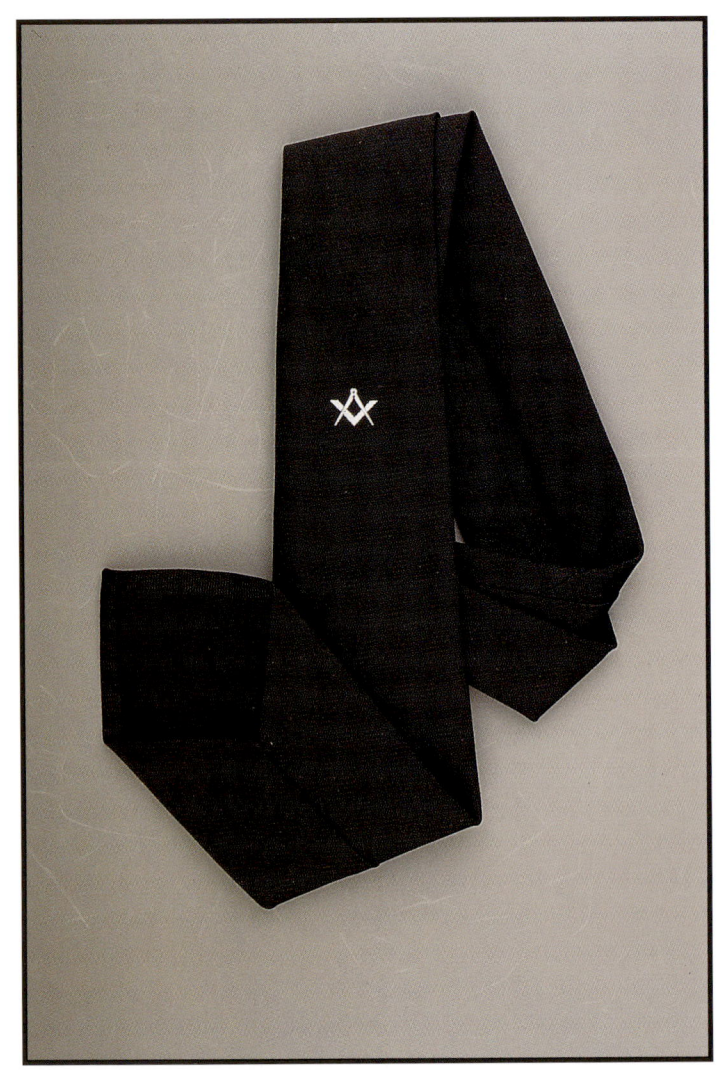

Masonic

100

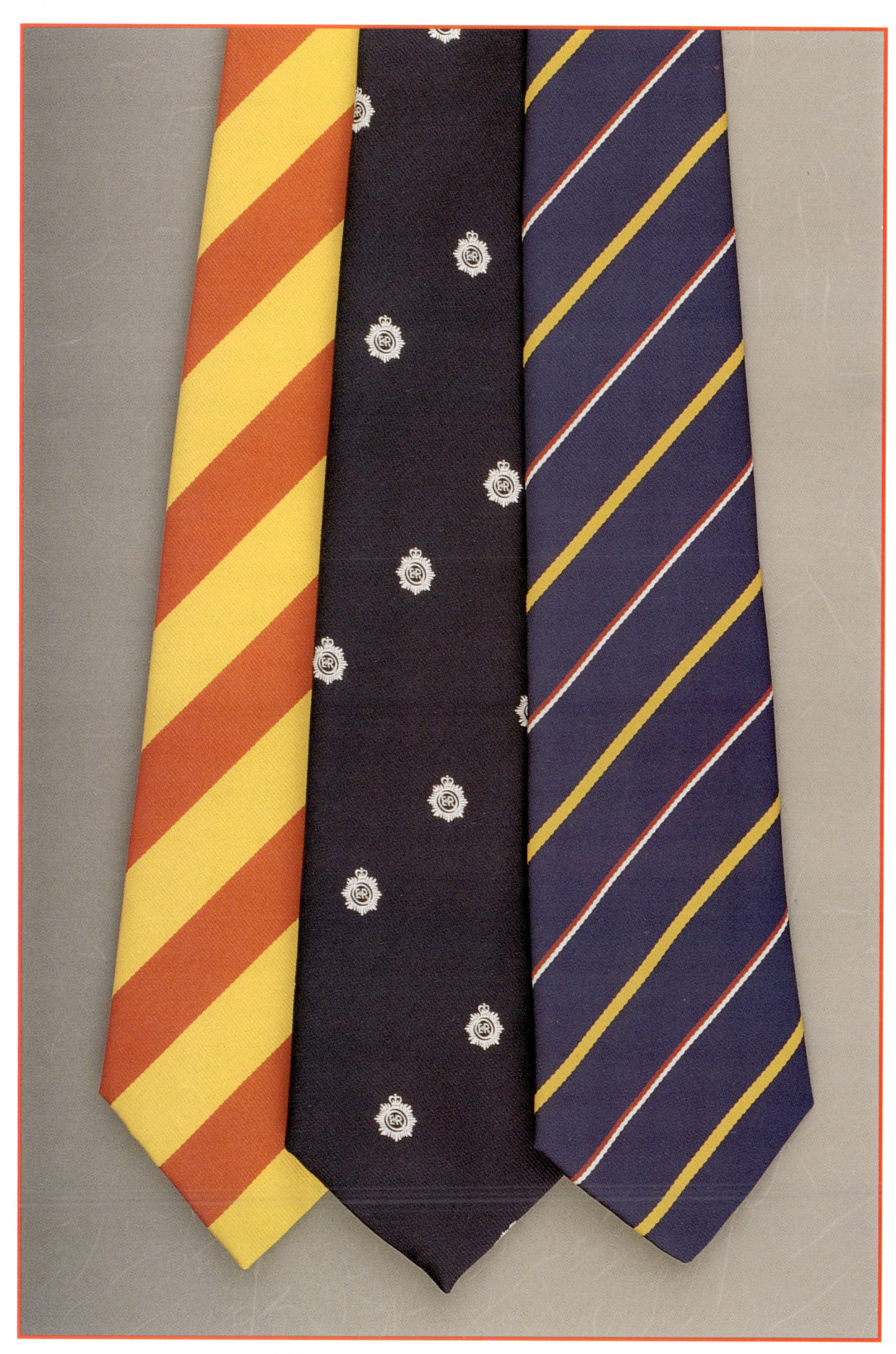

M.C.C.; Metropolitan Police; National Service

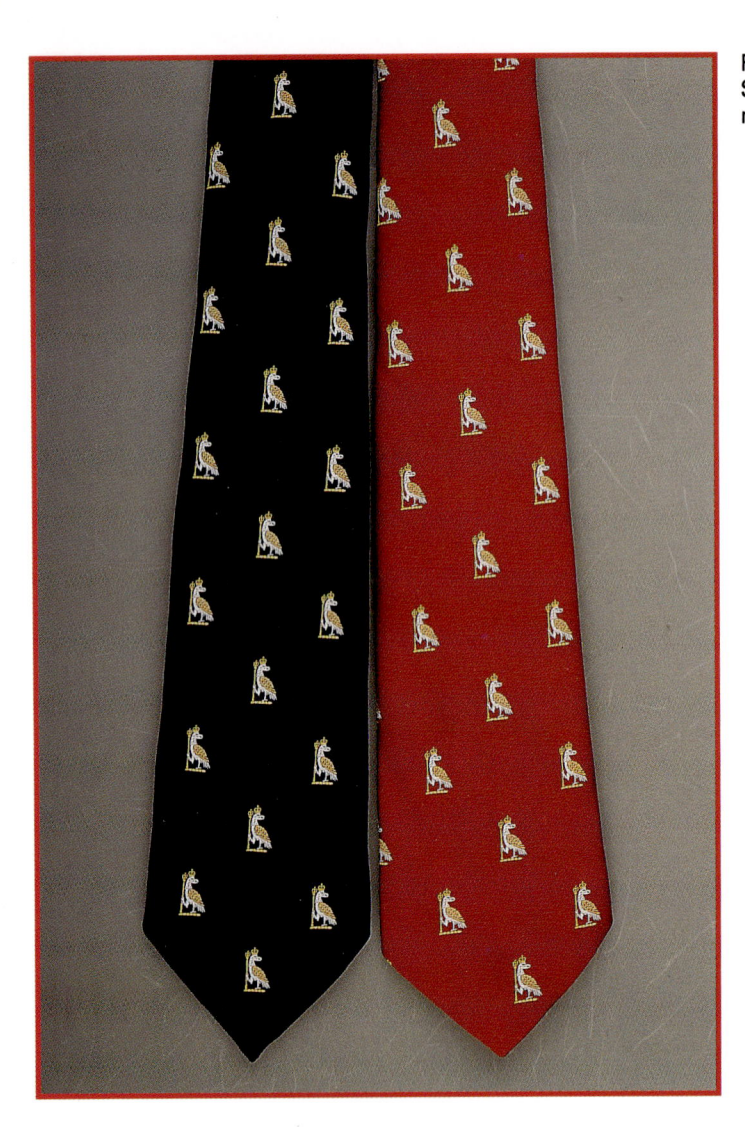

Royal College of Surgeons, navy and maroon grounds

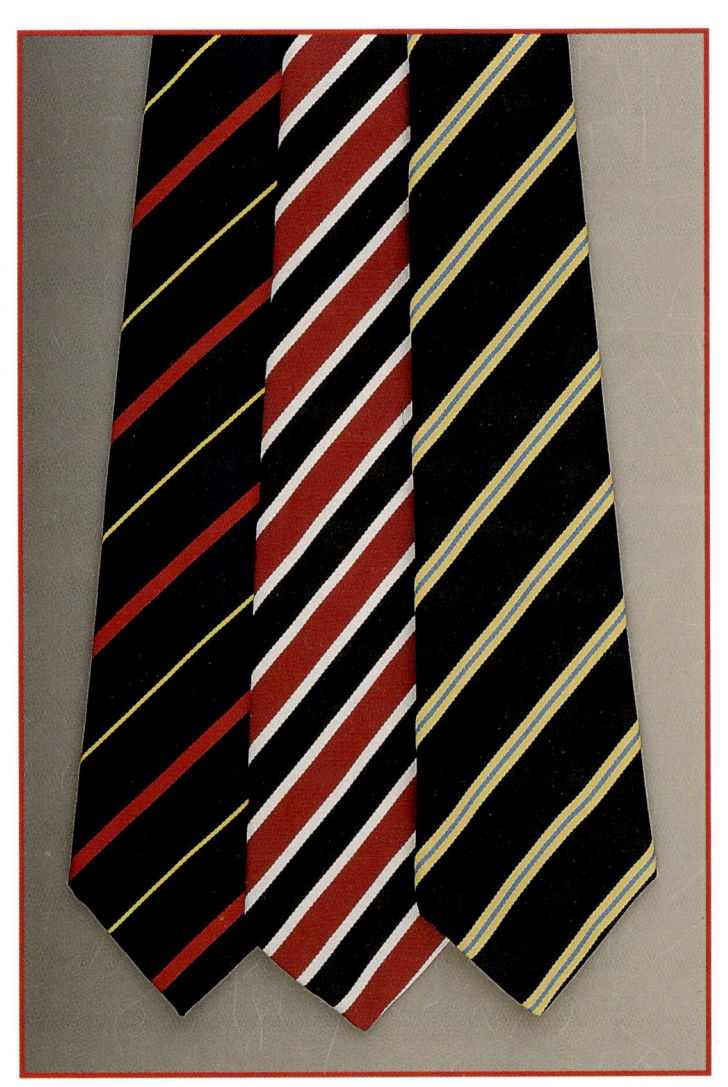

Trinity Field Club, Cambridge; Somerset County C.C.; Yorkshire County C.C.

102

National and County Ties

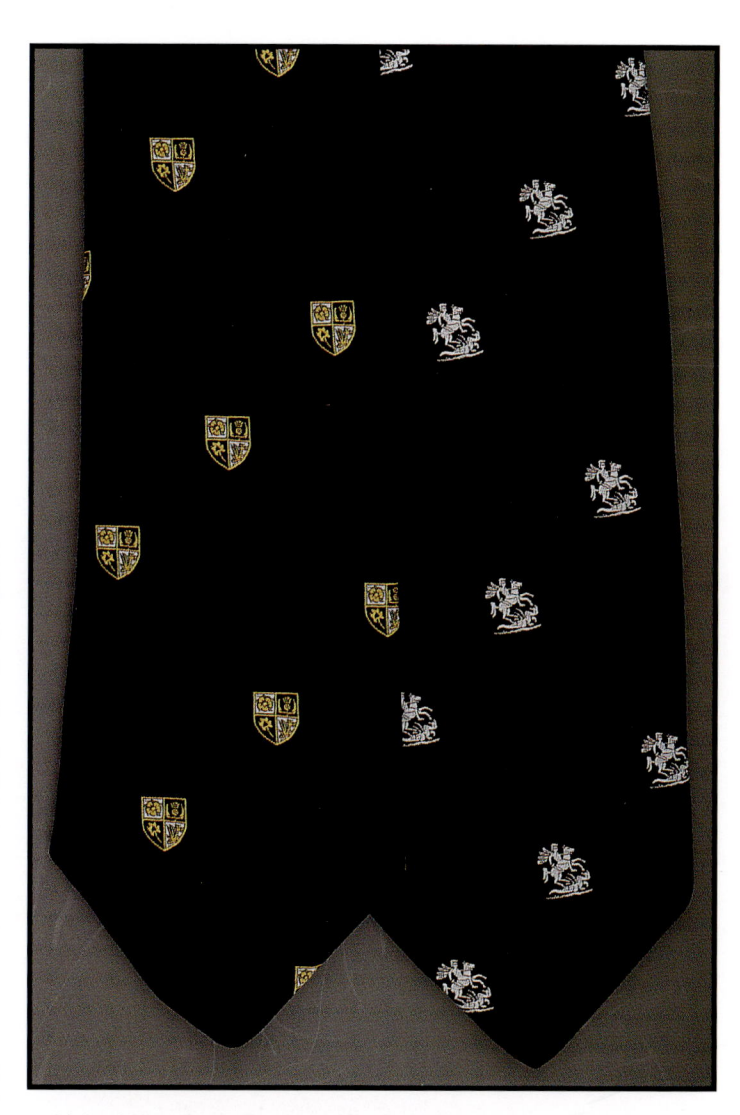

United Kingdom; England (St. George)

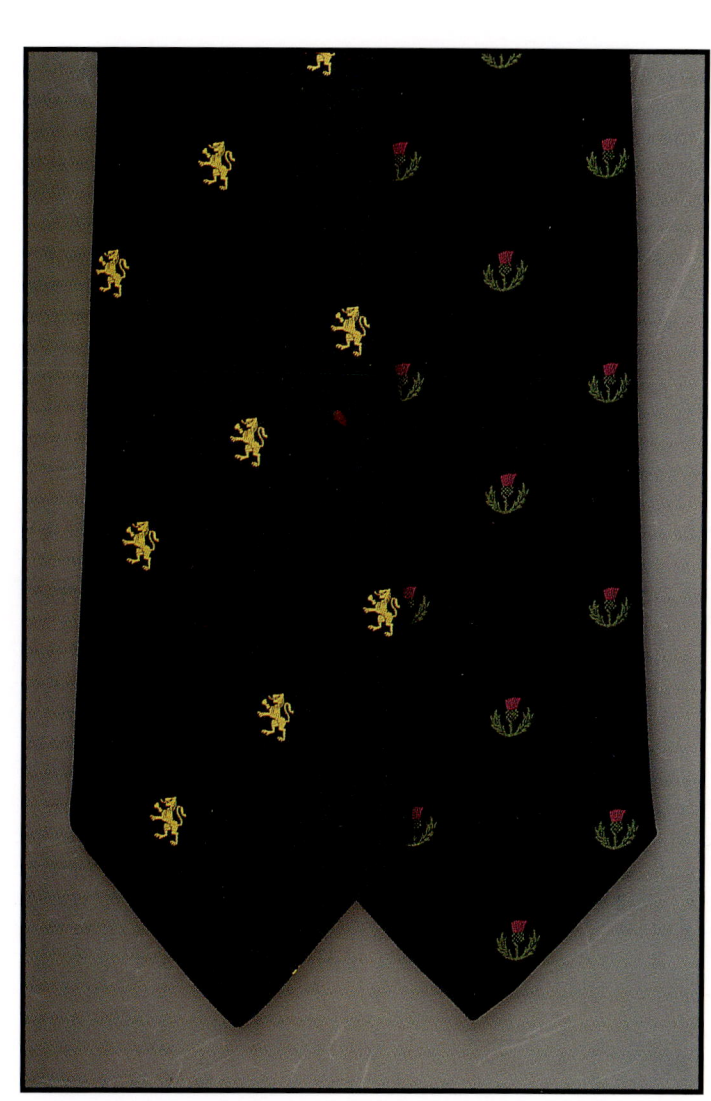

Scotland, lion and thistle

Wales; Ireland

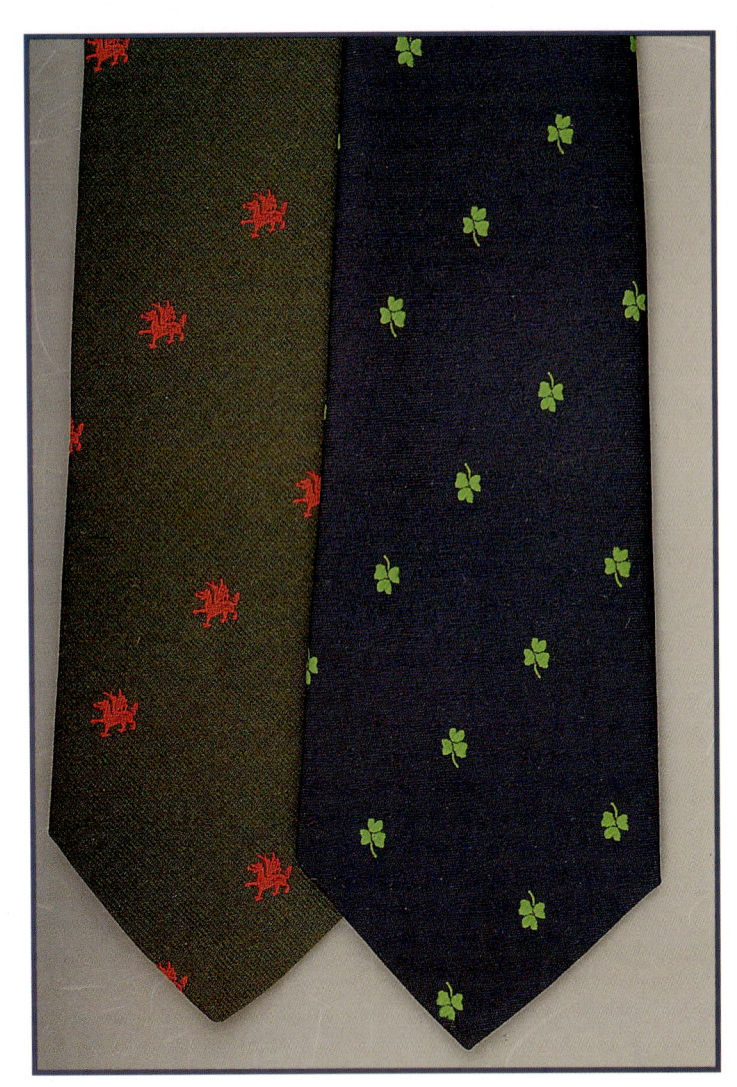

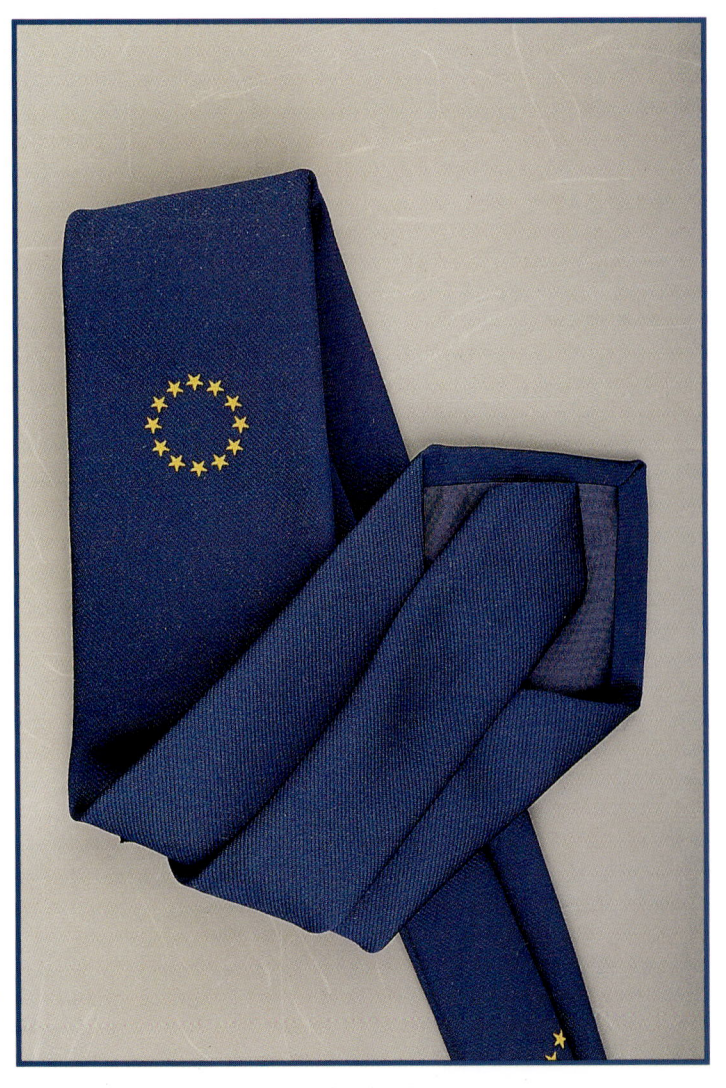

European Community

104

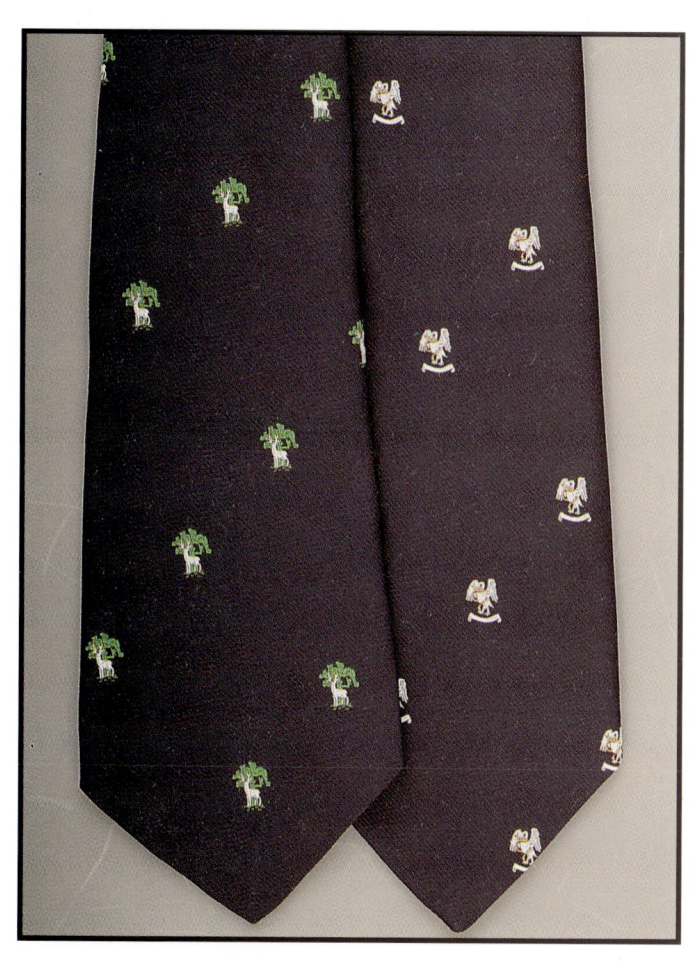

Berkshire; Buckinghamshire

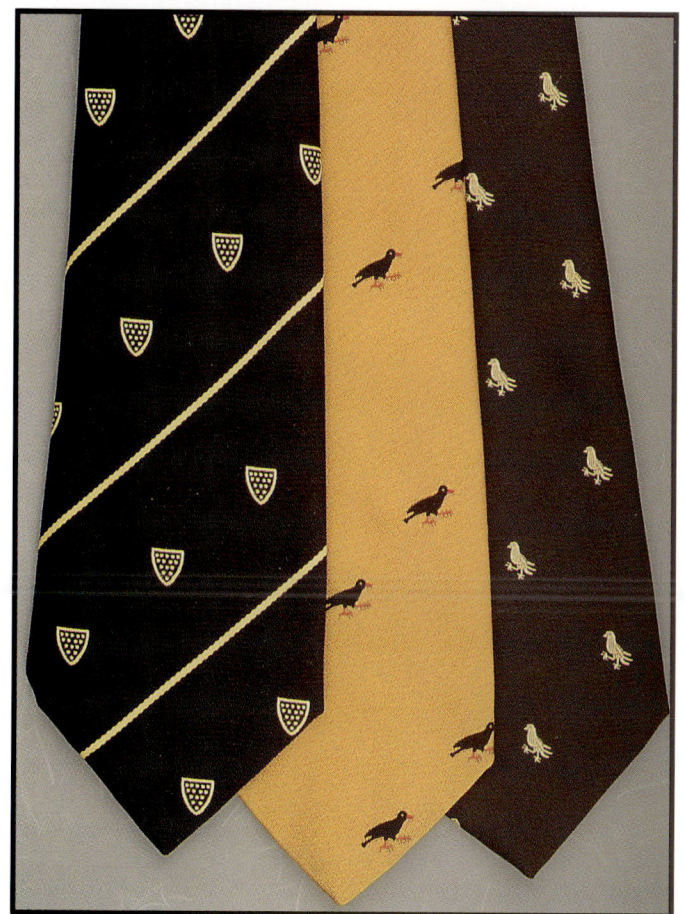

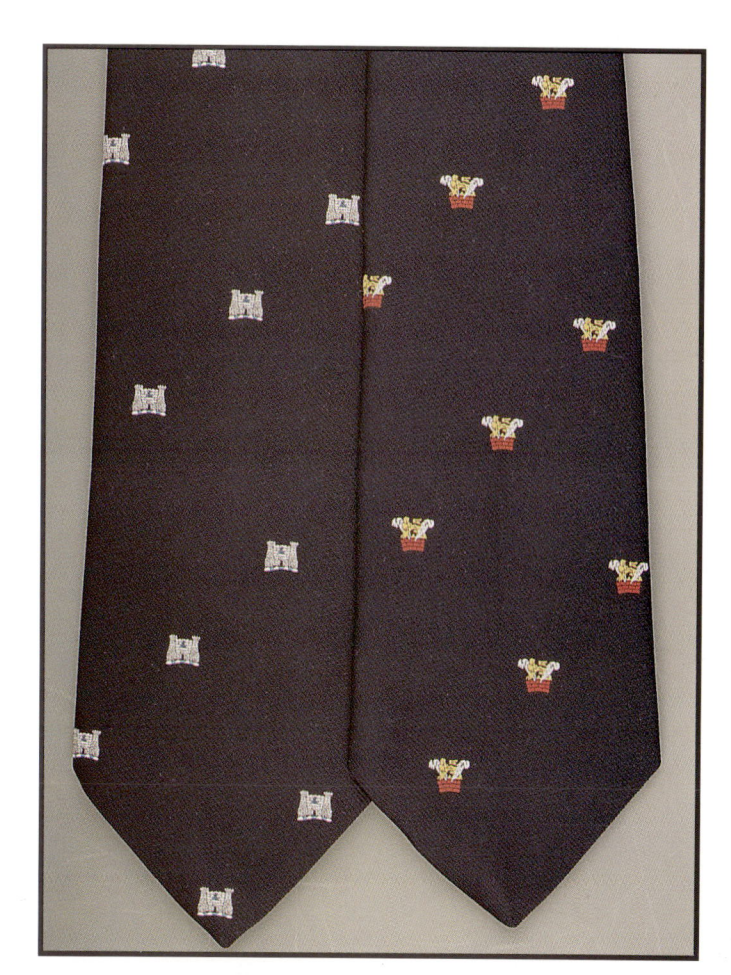

Cambridgeshire; Cheshire

Cornwall, crest and chough on gold and black

Derbyshire; Devonshire

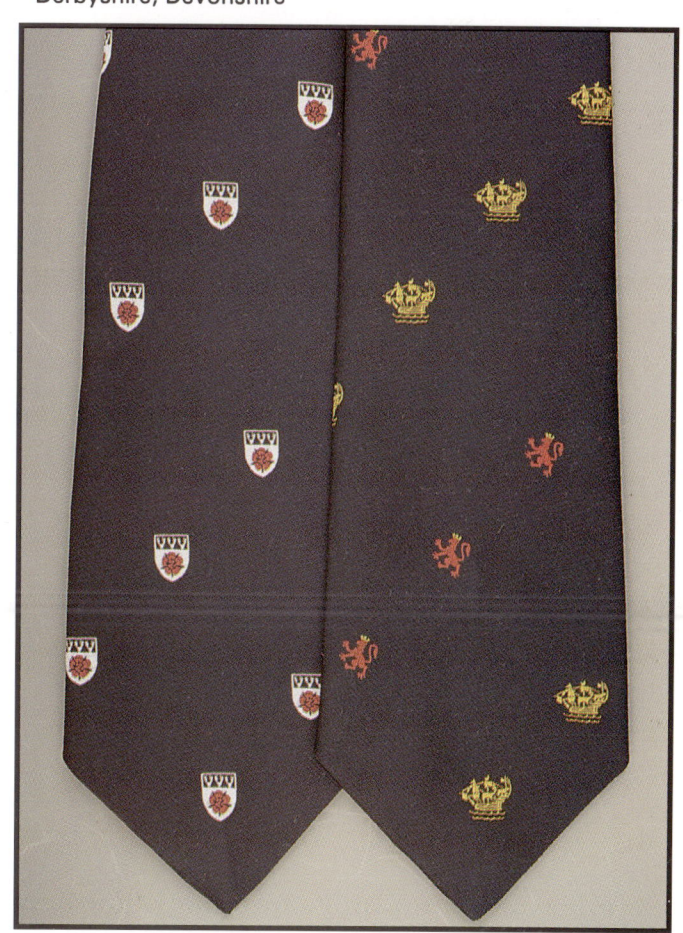

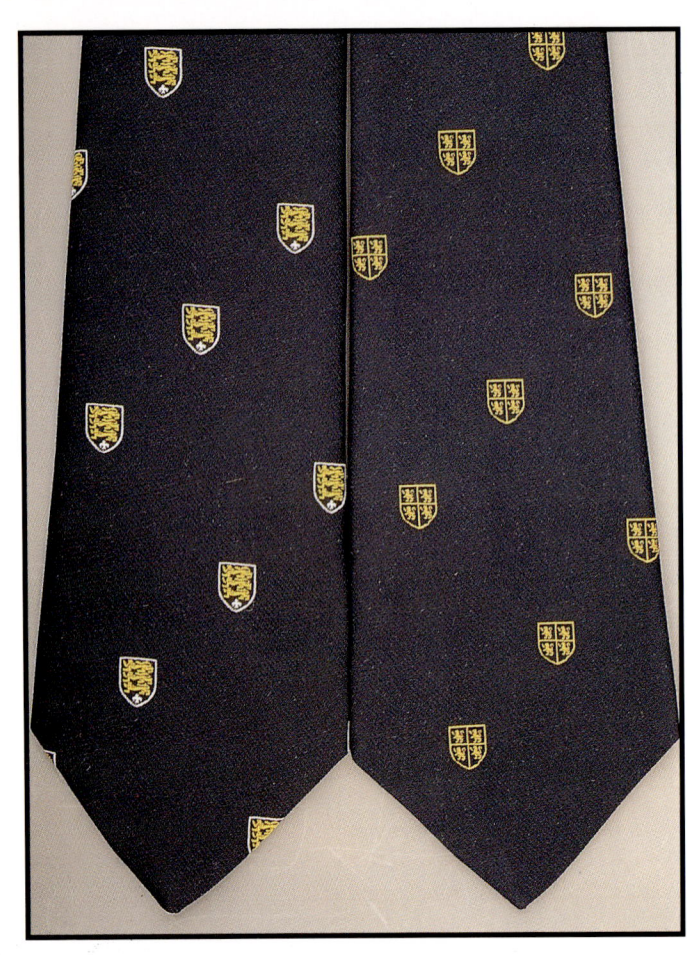

Dorset; Co. Durham

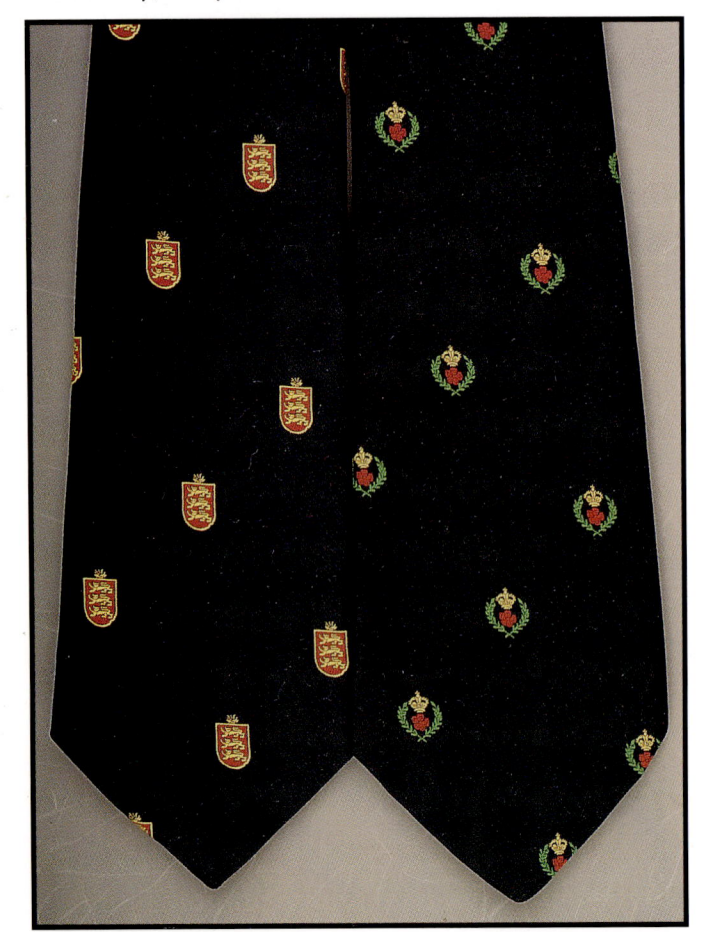

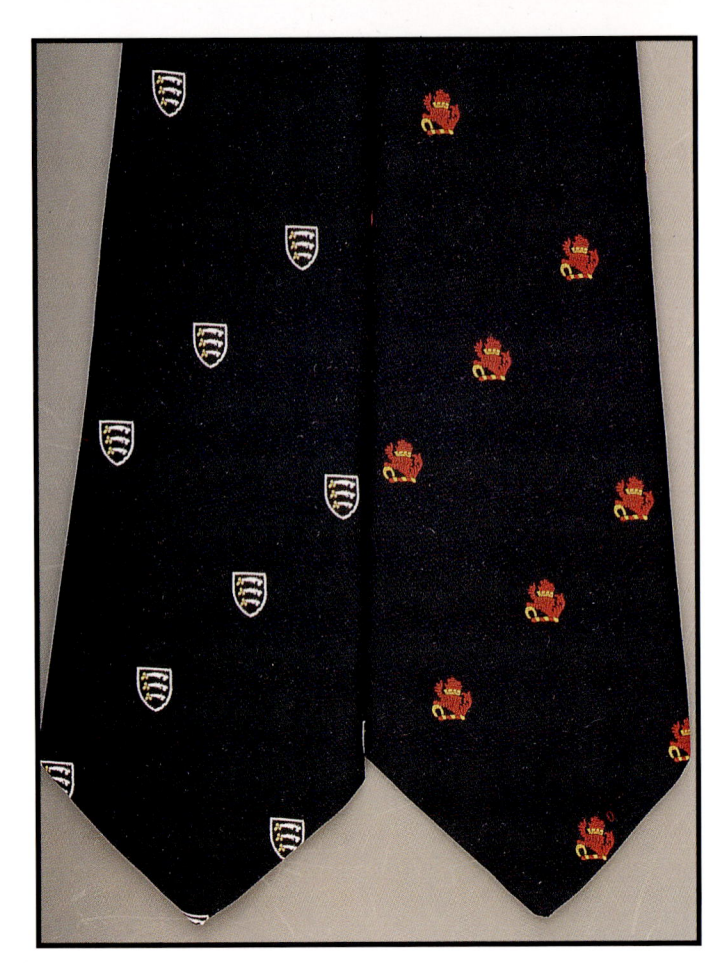

Essex; Gloucestershire

Guernsey; Hampshire

Herefordshire: Hertfordshire

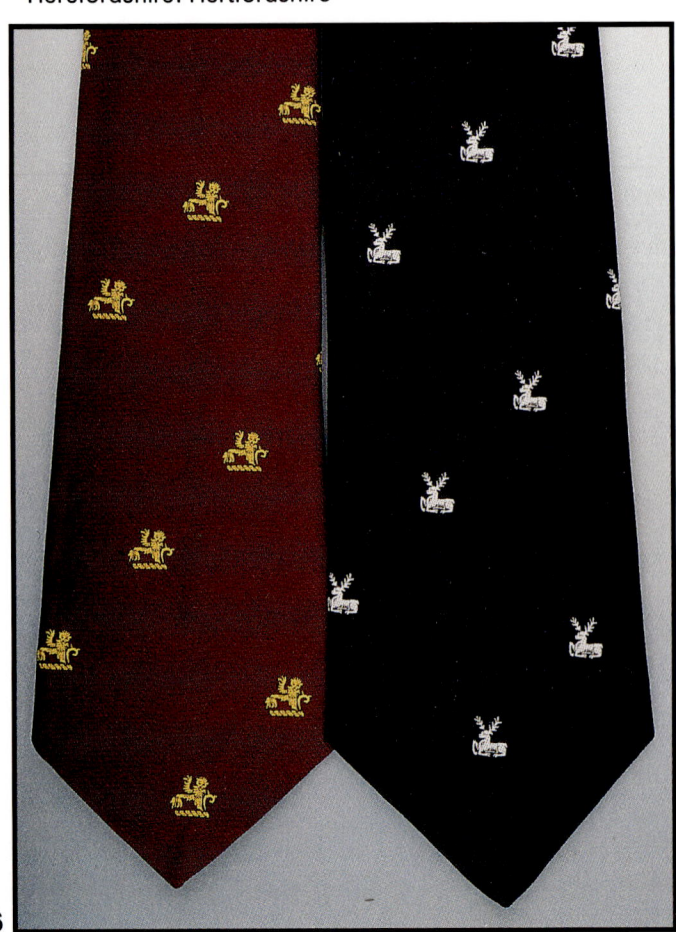

106

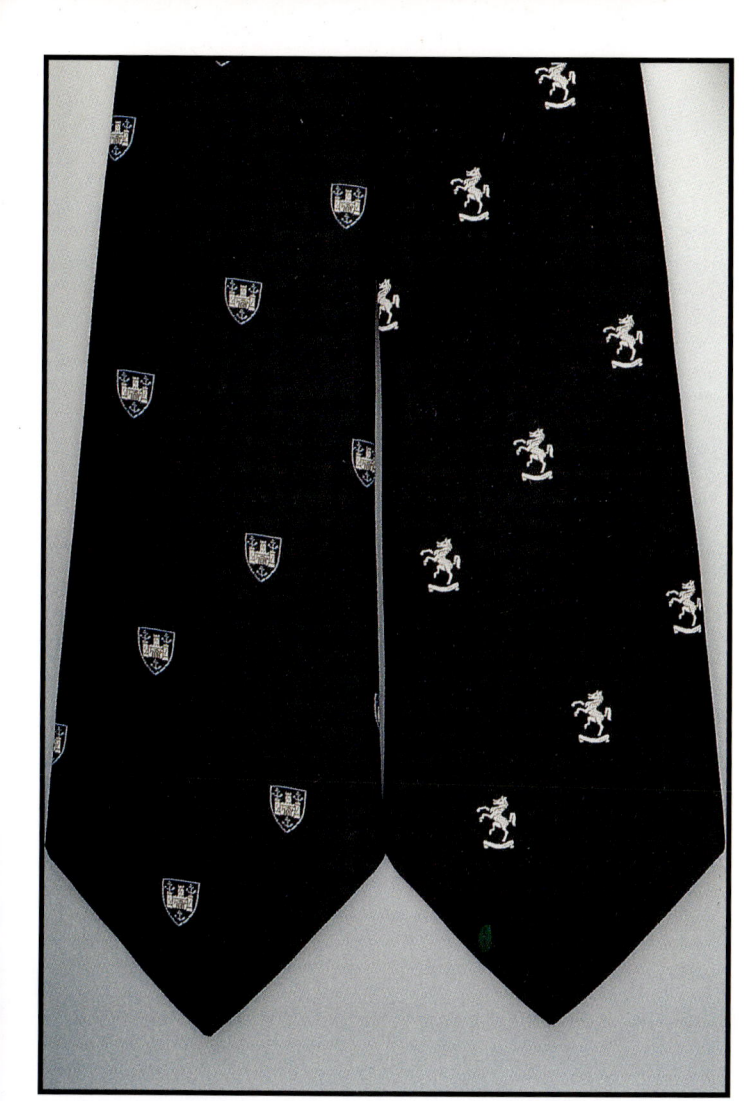

Isle of Wight; Kent

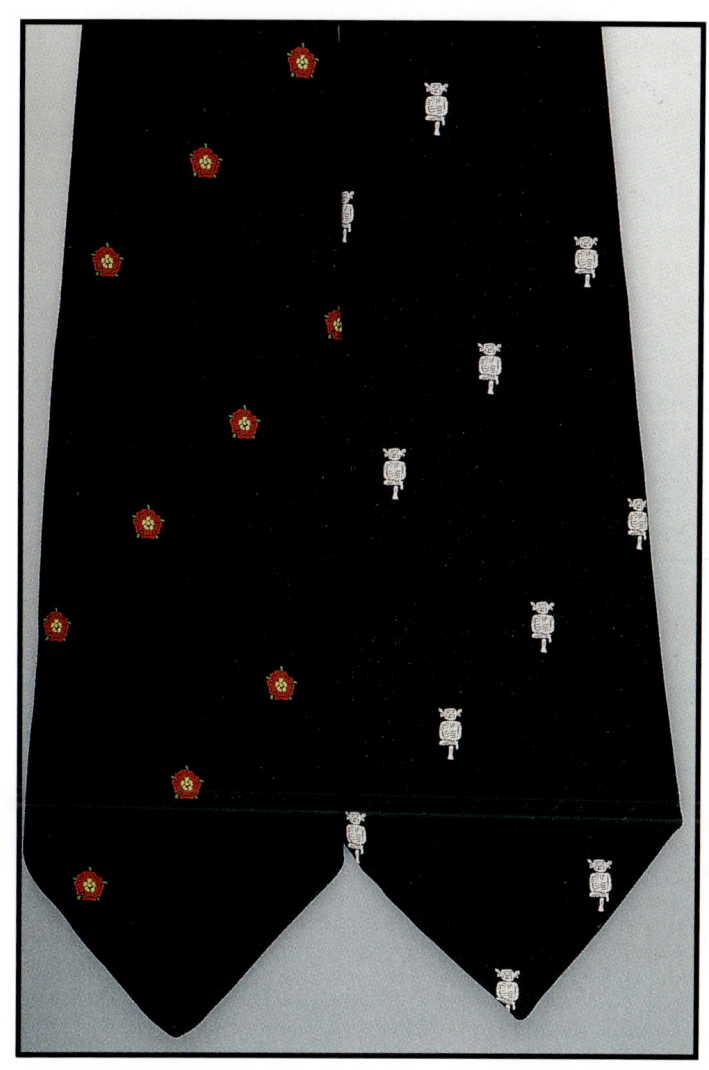

Lancashire;
Lincolnshire

107

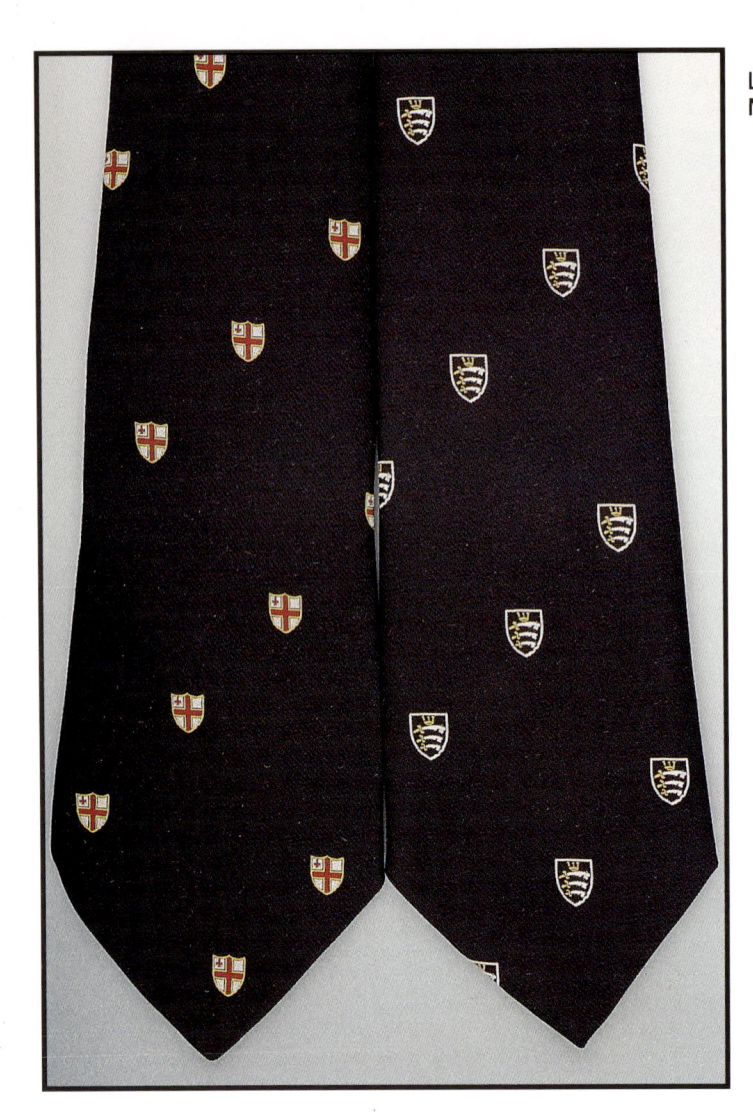

London;
Middlesex

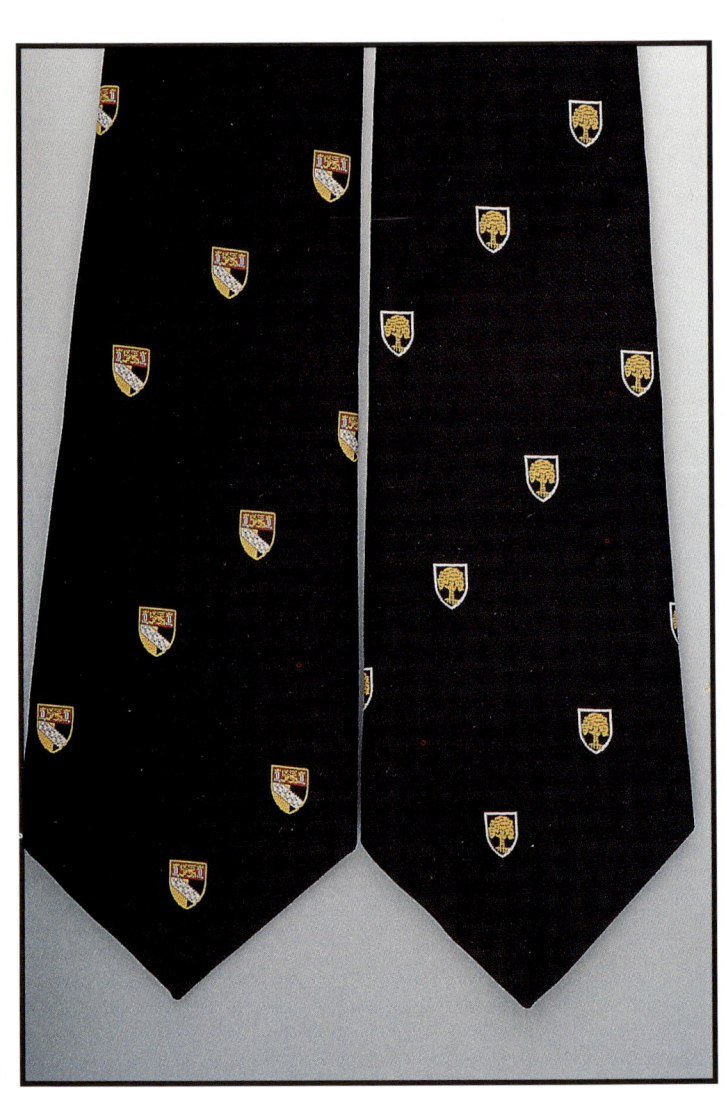

Norfolk;
Nottinghamshire

108

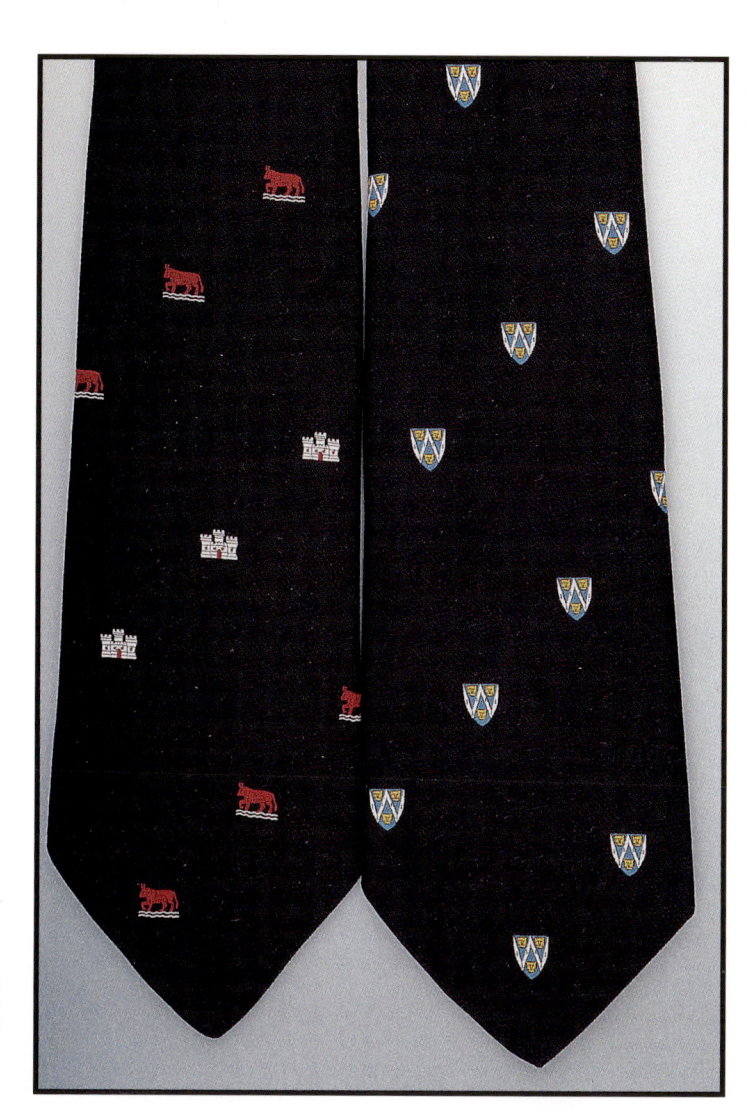

Oxfordshire;
Shropshire

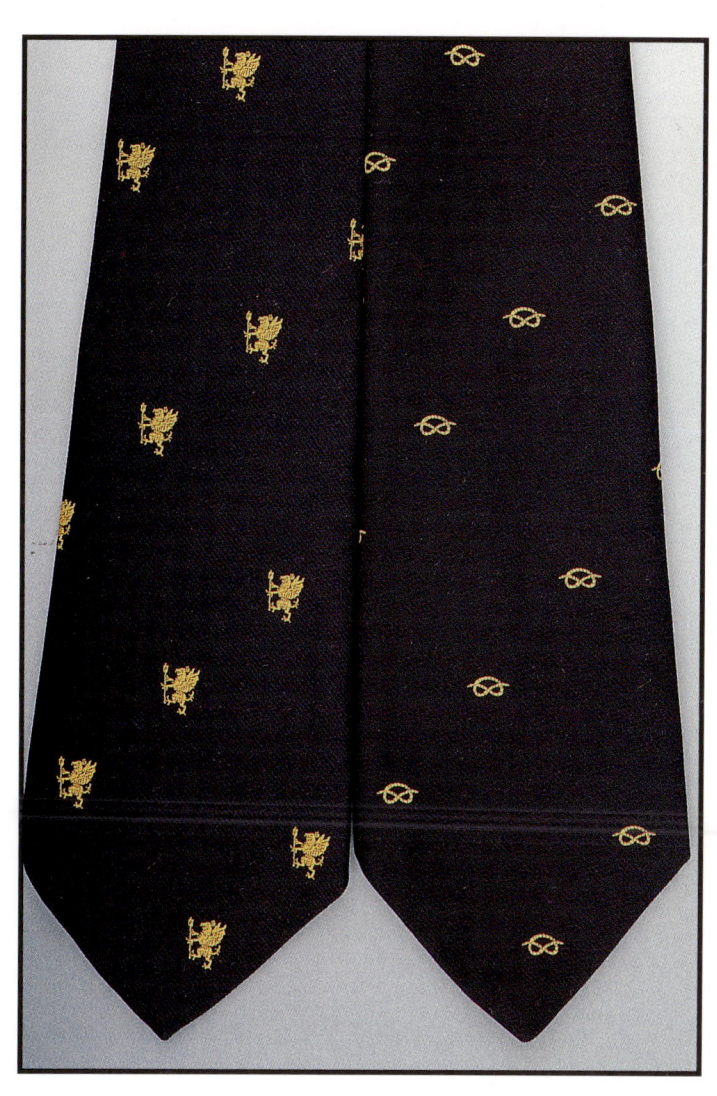

Somerset;
Staffordshire

Suffolk; Surrey

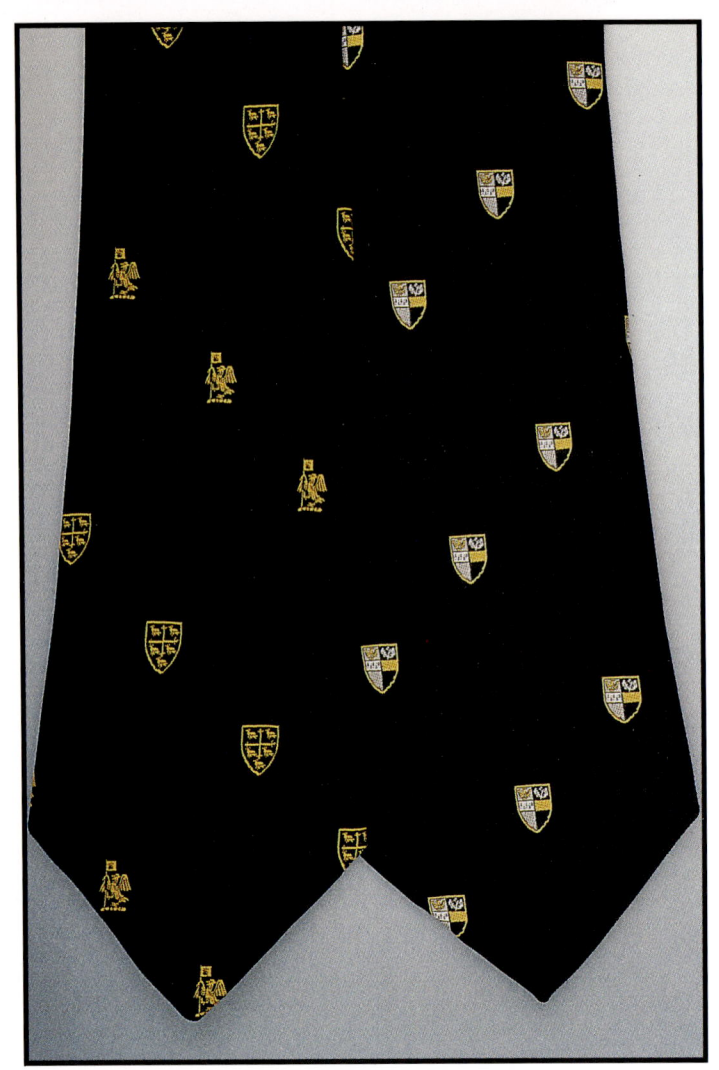

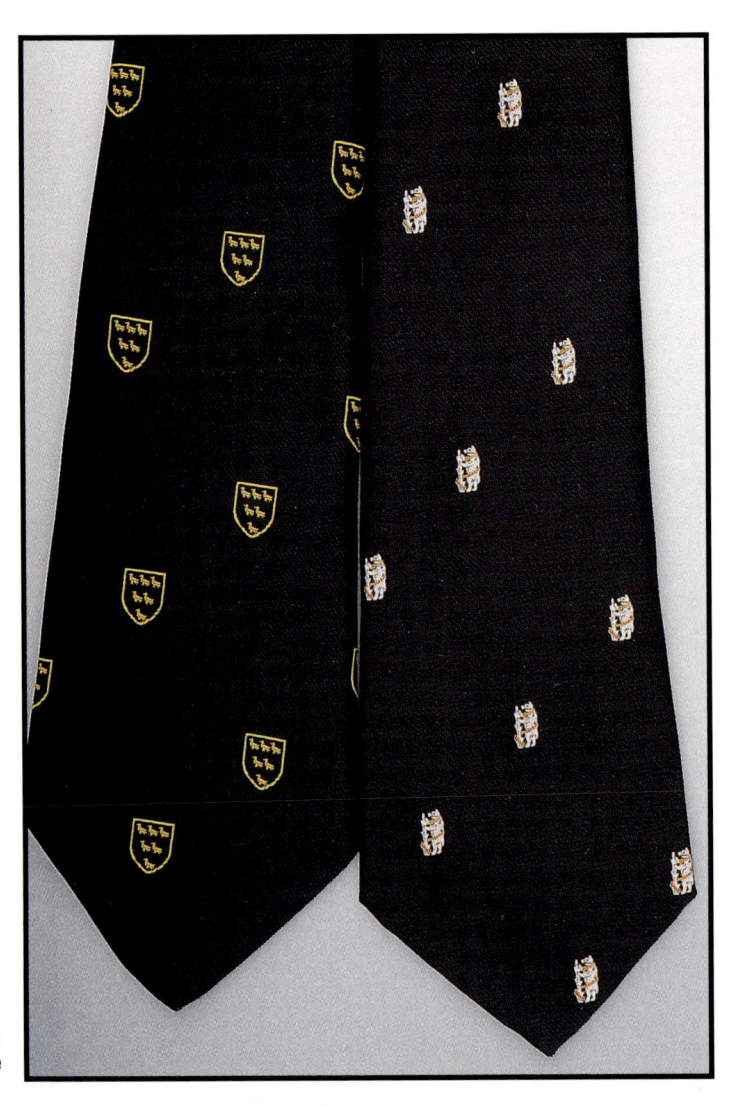

Sussex; Warwickshire

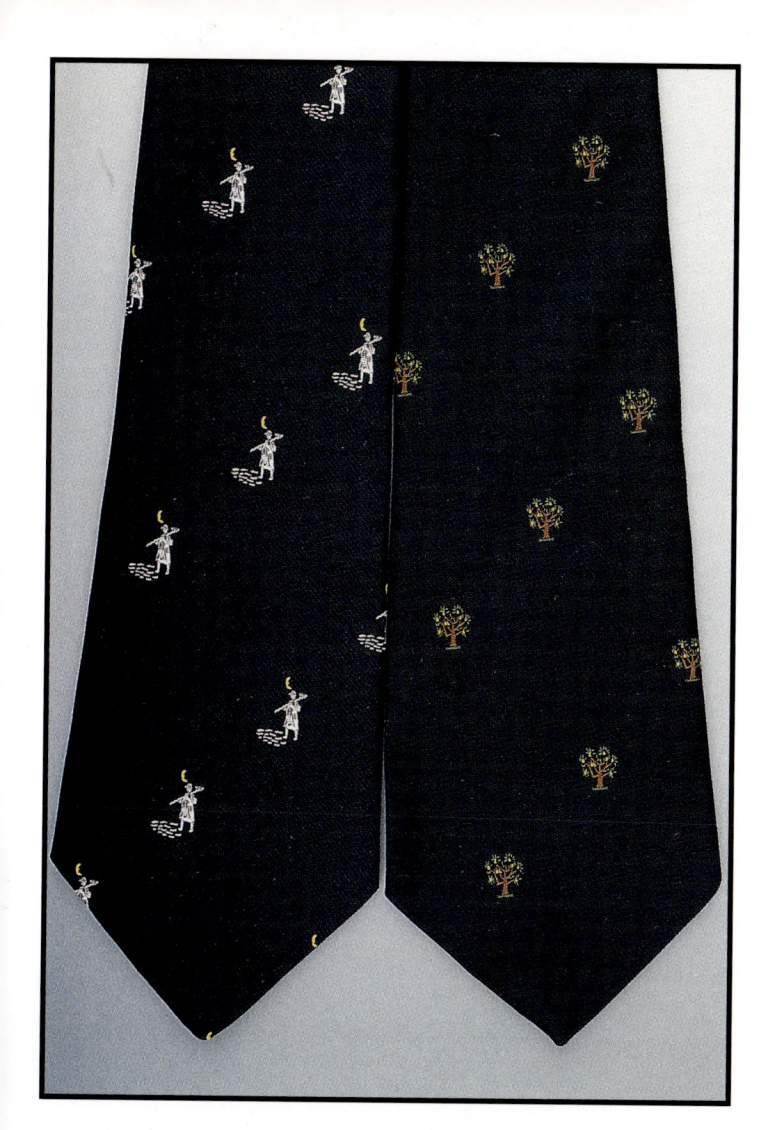

Wiltshire;
Worcestershire

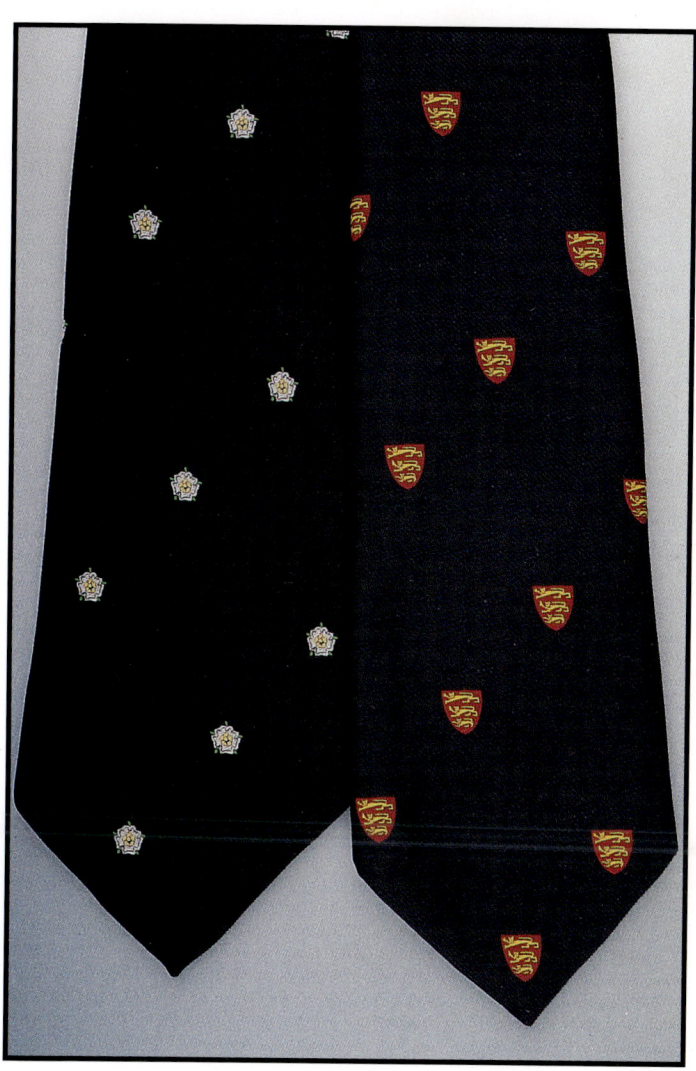

Yorkshire; Jersey
and England

111

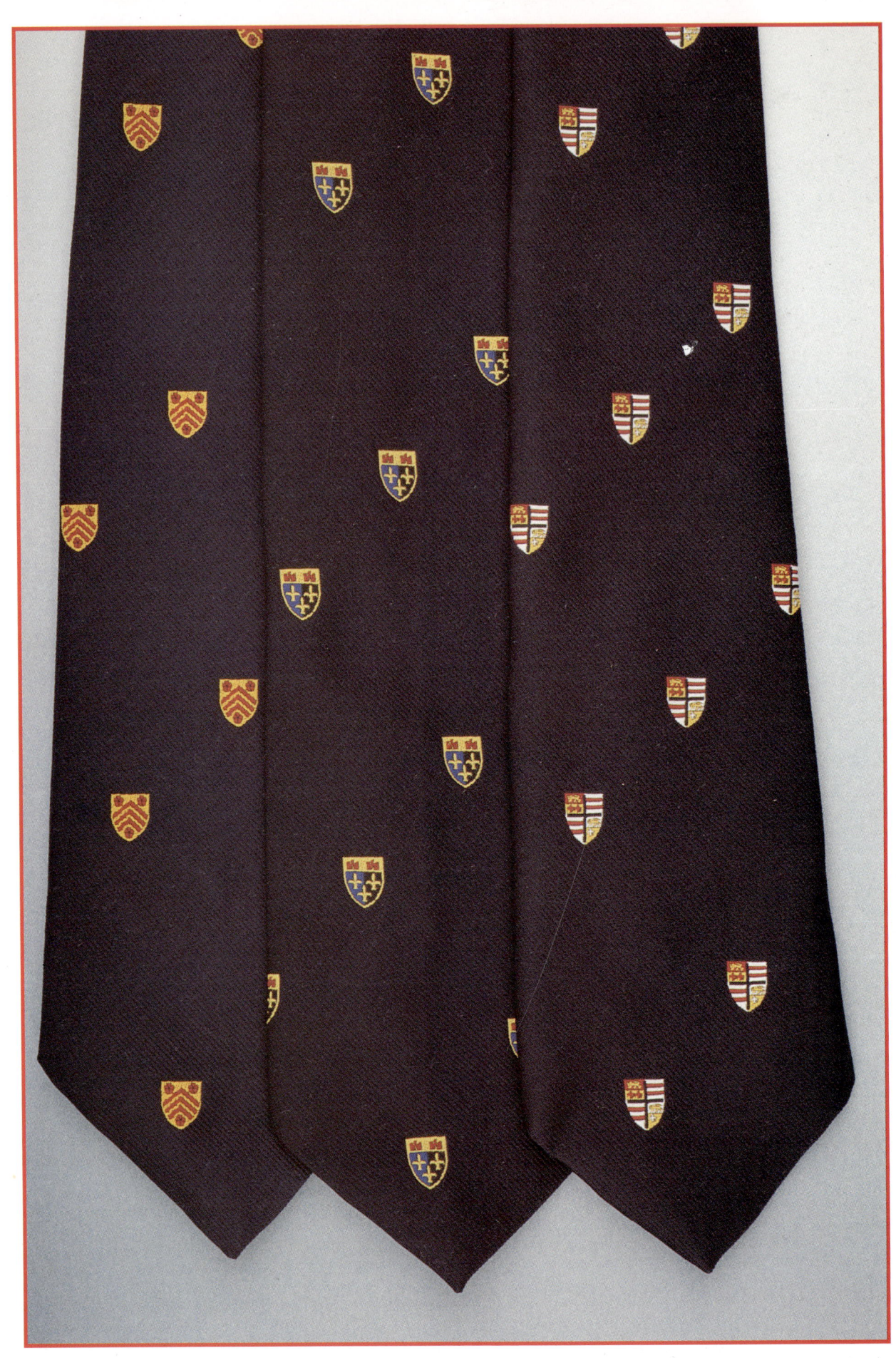

Glamorgan; Monmouthshire; Pembrokeshire